JOIN THE REVOLUTION!

A revolution has begun. Its drumbeats are echoing across the land—a call back to "live" foods and national health. Its banner is an apron, its weapons kitchen cutlery, and its soldiers an army of ex-junkies (junk food addicts) determined to kick the habit of bankrupt foods that are weakening and killing our generation.

The results of yesterday's poor dietary habits can't be totally overcome. But if you're ready to join the nutrition revolution, be prepared for some changes in your life. The withdrawal isn't all that bad.

HOW TO EAT RIGHT and FEEL GREAT

HOW TO EAT RIGHT and FEEL GREAT

Virginia
and
Norman
Rohrer

TYNDALE HOUSE PUBLISHERS
Wheaton, Illinois

Publisher's note: This book offers general nutritional guidelines toward physical and mental well being; the reader is advised to consult his personal physician for specific application of dietary principles to best fit individual needs and remedy specific ailments.

Cover illustration by Bonnie Nixon. Library of Congress Catalog Card Number 76-46042. ISBN 8423-1517-9, paper. Copyright © 1977 by Tyndale House Publishers, Inc., Wheaton, Illinois 60187. All rights reserved. Printed in the United States of America.

First printing, February 1977
Second printing, April 1977
Third printing, October 1977

To Don
for whom this book
came too late

Contents

Haven't you yet learned that your body is the home of the Holy Spirit God gave you, and that he lives within you? Your own body does not belong to you. For God has bought you with a great price. So use every part of your body to give glory back to God, because he owns it.

1 Corinthians 6:19, 20
The Living Bible

Foreword

Thousands of years ago a Chinese physician observed that the body's only source of energy was the air breathed and the food eaten. It is logical to assume that advanced enlightenment would make the air more pure and our food more nutritious. Unfortunately, precisely the opposite is true.

How refreshing, then, to have this common sense book showing how to find health in the midst of pollution by the simple, inexpensive, and appetizing technique of selective eating.

Today's advertising will lead you astray, while following the exhortations in this book will give your body maximum nourishment resulting in increased vigor and good health.

Throughout the forty-one years of my medical practice I have worked toward alleviating pain and halting the advance of disease. I have discovered, however, that susceptibility to disease is lessened and recuperation from it more rapid when the body has been sustained by good nutrition.

The body will heal itself only if the nutrients are available when it reaches out with its selective manipulation. That is the plan God instituted at Creation. A pantry full of balanced nutriments will help work cures beyond the physician's black bag. If attention is given to the first, the second will often not be needed.

The authors of this wide-ranging guidebook have increased its practicability by including delectable recipes appropriate to each subject discussed. They will prove to the most reluctant palate that nutrition is not a bore! Virginia Rohrer has personally developed each recipe. Her family and friends have enjoyed the delicious results.

Chapter nine, on chelation, provides an abundance of information on this relatively new procedure. Much evidence is in its favor; however, the reader should be apprised that it presently is considered to be in the experimental phase. Hopefully we can all look forward to documentation of profound positive results within the near future. I would also subscribe to a cautious use of herbs (chapter six) since copious amounts in certain situations could be toxic.

I have always encouraged my patients to eat a well-balanced diet, low in sugar, free of empty calories, and high in fiber. Now I shall direct them to this book which offers abundant proof concerning the merits of selecting and preparing nutritious food.

Virginia and Norman themselves are perhaps the best proof of their affirmations. They have had the courage to adopt this philosophy of life and the rewards are evident. What's more, they are attainable by all who heed the message of this book.

M. Louise Benefield, M.D.
Long Beach, California

Preface

Citizens of the Western world have grown fat, tired, and depressed. Physicians are dealing with a morass of preventable diseases resulting from stomachs loaded with processed, preserved, and pulverized food, stripped of nutrients.

Medical researchers have discovered that 50 percent of all cancer in male patients surveyed was linked to a lifetime of poor nutrition. The 258-page staff report released by the United States Senate Select Committee on Nutrition calls for legislation to promote nutrition education in a variety of ways.

"Our eating habits and the composition of our food have changed radically," the Senate committee chairman announced. "The threat is not beri beri, pellagra or scurvy. Rather, we face the more subtle, but also more deadly, reality of millions of Americans loading their stomachs with food which is likely to make them obese, to give them high blood pressure, to induce heart disease, diabetes and cancer—in short, to kill them.... We face the tragedy of

15

anemic children failing in school and repeating that pattern of failure throughout their shortened lives."

An exhaustive three-year research project involving the United States Department of Agriculture, and several universities and land grant colleges, showed that nutrition alone was able to reduce the incidence of many common diseases and inadequate health *up to 80 percent.*

"The facts are in," stated Howard C. Long, president of the American Physical Fitness Institute of Los Angeles. "Sound nutrition does have a dramatic and lasting effect on health. Lifelong habit patterns are being established in youth and it is the time to provide them with guidance using current, scientific, motivating information on nutrition."

Organized medicine, as we have known it for so long, admits that drugs and the surgical knife are not alpha and omega; that preventive measures through nutrition are both possible and much to be preferred.

Dr. Sam E. Roberts, of the University of Kansas Medical School, makes the charge that "the medical students of the past who are our physicians today were taught little or nothing of nutrition and even less of deficiencies and imbalances."

Medical school curricula are largely preoccupied with diagnosis and specific therapy. Little time and attention are given to the nutritional aspects of therapeutics.

Alan H. Nittler, M.D., states in his book, *A New Breed of Doctor,* that at least 20 percent of hospitalized patients are there for treatment of iatrogenic diseases (those inadvertently caused by physicians or the drugs they prescribed). "This is a ridiculous record," Dr. Nittler adds.[1]

The traditional factors used to analyze diseases today are the patient's (1) age, (2) sex, (3) occupation, (4) residence, (5) past history, (6) family history, (7) heredity, and (8) stress. This leaves only one remaining frontier to explore and to consider: the nutritional profile of a patient, past, present, and future.

Citizens are ready for the change. They are open to the claims of the "healing" foods, which include deliverance from crippling disease, fatigue, depression, and obesity. They are ready for "live" foods, free from a deluge of sugar, fats, and chemicals. The ranks of nutrition enthusiasts are growing.

Prejudice against pioneering methods in nutrition is often only resistance to the extremists, not to the concept of giving the body what it needs to function best.

Classical medical practice has made tremendous strides in the control of disease, in the discovery of immunizations, and in the development of life-saving surgical procedures. The nutrition revolution is putting the spotlight on a new and more exciting preventive measure: good food.

Personal Words ...

From Virginia: As a little girl I learned a tune that pretty well sums up the attitude of my brother and sisters toward our mother's early zeal for a nutritious spread:

> Blackstrap molasses and wheat-germ bread,
> You'll live so long you'll wish you were dead.

But Mama would just smile at our teasing and keep brewing her herbs, steaming her grains, and mastering the art of waterless cooking. She raised a quartet of pink-cheeked youngsters who never needed to see a medical doctor throughout the two decades of their minority (except for a mastoid operation for my brother).

I began to take food supplements as a teen-ager in high school. The exhilaration of good health was my constant companion. Nutrition has been a part of my study and practice since, and I think we have evidence in our family that bushels of tasty prevention are surely worth more than even a spoonful of cure. It ought to be said often: Every drug "cure" has a side effect or a contraindication.

We are hopeful that the knowledge we have gained from research and personal experience will give you a more radiant and abundant life. He who has health has a God-given blessing no riches can buy.

From Norman: They don't come any healthier than the German farmers of Pennsylvania's Lancaster County. I should know. I was one of them. I thought that the nutritional legacy of my farm heritage and the bounty of fresh farm produce had prepared me for anything, but I was wrong.

When I chose a career in writing and editing, I entered into a stressful occupation which took a heavy toll in my health, leading to hypoglycemia, allergies, and other annoying results of deadline pressures.

But a new day has dawned for me, thanks to my wife's persistence in exploring the possibilities of nutrition. We're still learning, but it's pleasurable to enjoy blessed, ongoing, unmedicated relief. It's fun to feel good again. With me it has become a spiritual issue. The person who knows how to eat nutritionally and doesn't, I believe that to him it is sin.

We hope that these case histories, statistics, and miscellaneous collection of a hundred and one nutritional tips will contribute to the health and happiness of you and your loved ones.

Virginia and Norman Rohrer

CHAPTER ONE

What's So Great About Nutrition

Tell me what you eat and I will tell you what you are.
—Brillat Savarin, *Physiologie du Gout*

A spindly teen-ager stepped to the counter of a southern California fast-food restaurant and placed his usual order for lunch: "A coke and large fries."

It was 12:15 P.M. His afternoon high school schedule still held an examination in French, a forty-five minute algebra class, and gym.

The young man bolted his lunch as he drove back to campus. His only other fortification that day had been five teaspoons of sugar, a stab of caffeine, and a dash of salt and fat. (For breakfast that morning he had had a donut and a cup of coffee.)

That evening at home he became sullen and irritable, too tired to finish his homework and too upset to eat the dinner his mother had prepared. To each suggestion that he eat, he reacted curtly. He seemed eager to quarrel with his father and defensive about his plans for the evening.

19

Before dinner was over he left the house, hurling a barrage of verbal abuse at his parents. Close to midnight the parents were notified that their son had led the police on a high-speed chase and had failed to turn a corner. He had crashed into a cement retaining wall and was lacerated severely as he was thrown from the hurtling car.

Was diet to blame for this erratic behavior? There may have been other contributing influences, but our research convinces us that food, or lack of it, definitely affects our moods.

An Indianapolis businessman directed a growing distributing company for precision tools. But as his responsibilities grew he found less and less energy for keeping pace with the challenges of his expanding business. Checkups at a famous clinic revealed nothing organically wrong. The man gorged himself with carbohydrates to try to keep up his energy, adding unsightly pounds and further frustrations.

In a fit of depression he abruptly left the church in which he and his family had once been happy. He became jealous of his wife, who was active in community projects. His mental vacillation and physical languor caused psychological distortions. He punished his children too severely and became petulant and moody.

He was a victim of outrageous eating habits which were obvious to even the most casual observer. Yet when the businessman was tested at a local hospital and treated for pancreatitis the physicians and specialists neither mentioned diet nor inquired about his eating habits. Their advice was simply: "Don't drink any alcoholic beverages." Alcohol was not a problem to the patient.

Later, when his pancreatitis grew worse, he was admitted to a prestigious Midwestern medical clinic. Again, the doctors neither said anything about his diet nor cautioned him against eating an almost-exclusively carbohydrate diet. At the age of thirty-eight the young father died in his sleep of arteriosclerosis. A reduction of carbohydrates and a balanced diet could have saved his life.

For six years an eastern Pennsylvania news reporter had endured a burning sensation in his bladder which puzzled doctors and worried his family.

"Don't come in again until you take a two-week vacation," one doctor advised. The newsman did better. He took his family to the World's Fair in Japan and spent an entire month relaxing in the Orient. Still the pain persisted.

"You have interstitial cystitis," another urologist said, following an extensive diagnosis. "Take these tranquilizers four times a day. There is no cure, only occasional relief by filling the bladder with silver nitrate. We really don't know altogether why this helps, but it seems to."

The newsman faithfully took the pills until their effect wore off and the burning returned. He had to rise as many as five times a night to empty his bladder to relieve the pain.

After he was given an intravenous pyelogram, the patient was told by still another doctor that the pressure of deadlines kept his bladder tender. In desperation, the newsman asked for an entire year's leave of absence from his job, rented his house, and moved his family to a cabin in the mountains. But still the cure eluded him.

After six years and six specialists, he returned home puzzled and discouraged. One day he heard a nurse casually remark that wheat is near the top among annoying allergens which plague people in a variety of ways. He stopped eating wheat and found blessed, dramatic relief within a week.

What's so great about nutrition? Rather a lot, we think. What you eat governs how you act, how you look, and how you feel. Nutrition is more than liquefied grass, stone-ground eggs, and bitter herbs. Good nutrition can help the body build and heal itself, experience relief from pain, fortify itself against fatal diseases, and avoid mental and emotional disorders. When you feed the body wholesome foods free from sugar and chemical saturation it soon loses its taste for the artificial.

The science of nutrition is exploding. Empty foods are in trouble. Yesterday we spoke in terms of "minimum daily requirements." Tomorrow we are going to eat to *stay well* through "maximum daily requirements" that will make trips to doctors' offices less frequent. You will enjoy the fulfillment of glowing health and sharpened mental capabilities. You will enjoy diets that banish fatigue and offer added stamina. In short, you will help your body to do its job with "high octane fuel" at the table.

"Why didn't my doctor tell me?"

There are no finer, more dedicated professional people than physicians. We look to them for diagnoses and prescriptions when we are ill. It is unfair to expect medical and surgical doctors also to have mastered the vast science of nutrition.

Twenty years ago not one medical school in the United States offered a course in nutrition. When we asked our gynecologist how much time he had spent in nutritional training he replied, "I had none."

A heart specialist told us candidly, "I finished my training with three diets: One for low-sodium requirements, one for reducing, and one for diabetics."

Generally, what little nutrition is taught concerns itself with the recognition of deficiency diseases such as beri beri, pellagra, or scurvy—diseases which rarely exist today. Patients are often misled and sometimes allowed to suffer needlessly when good food and an altered diet could do much to restore their health.

The United States spends more than $100 billion each year seeking health, yet in comparison with other countries, it comes off poorly in many categories—deaths, drug dependence, accidents, and alcoholism.

Calling for preventive measures rather than curative treatment, Dr. Halfdan T. Mahler, Director-General of the World Health Organization, criticized the practice of giving first place to curative medicine and second to the prevention of disease and promotion of health.

"Healthy families make healthy people," he stated in the September 1975 issue of *World Health* magazine. "Yet in many parts of the world today the medical establishments, obsessed as they are with a concern for marginal disease, are doing far from enough to provide health care for the family." Instead, Dr. Mahler declared, "Vast technological resources are deployed to cope with a small number of 'sophisticated' diseases while the prevention of disease and promotion of health definitely take second place."

He regretted that in developing countries the practice of the Western world is being duplicated. "The same kind of dependence on the health professional and his drugs is being fostered with regrettable energy. And to make the situation worse, these countries are also forsaking sound traditional practices, as for instance breast-feeding."

He also said that much of what was sound in the traditional practices of the past is being destroyed in the name of progress—not only through inevitable social change, but also as a result of "downright profiteering and misguided professionalism." Such radical changes in family health care, however, will "depend upon the health professional to listen to the needs and desires of the people," he said.

In a report by the Select Committee on Nutrition and Human Needs of the U.S. Senate, recognition of malnutrition and its aftermath was given: "Malnutrition appears to be the common denominator in each of these problems—low birth weight, infant mortality, mental retardation and intellectual malfunction. Any attempt to break the cycle of poverty characterized by these phenomena must include intervention or this waste of human life will continue unabated."

A research report prepared by Dr. Paul Podmajersky for the convention in Las Vegas of the American Society of Bariatric Physicians (obesity specialists) stated that only 24 percent of America's adults can be considered "normal" with regard to weight and blood pressure. The other 76 percent grouping, Dr. Podmajersky said, "is either overweight, has high blood pressure or both." His study contradicts the figures previously given in accepted surveys on the national statistical average for weight and blood pressure.

The state of our nation's health is deteriorating. The chemical pollution of both environment and food is taking a heavier toll than we imagined. A medical bulletin recently released states that 80 percent of the incidents of cancer in the United States are the result of this outrageous pollution.

A nutrition revolution must begin now. It must begin in your kitchen and ours. Each of us has emotional reasons for disliking certain foods and liking others. Go easy on your family. Make changes gradually. Introduce a disliked-but-healthful food with a favorite. Request that each member taste the new dish to get acquainted. Variety will provide a more healthful life.

So, What's Great About Nutrition?

It contributes to mental stability.

Most people eat without thinking about their body's most important organ—the brain. Poor nutrition can weaken the brain's ability to control bodily functions and lead to unstable emotional behavior as well. (See chapter two.)

It overcomes today's chemical scourge.

More than half the foods you buy in your supermarket are prepackaged, preserved, and processed—great for long shelf life, but who wants to eat dead food? The result of eating sugar- and chemical-saturated foods is of little consequence in small doses. But ingested over a long period? (See chapter three.)

It produces better babies.

The first eighteen months in a child's growth and development, beginning at conception, are critical. They determine largely the child's health, mental capacity, and fulfillment. The United States ranks fourteenth in cases of infant mortality and eighteenth on graphs showing life expectancy for male babies.

It is never too early for a future mother to prepare for her baby's birth with the help of body-building nutrition. (See chapter four.)

It fortifies against allergies.

There is more to allergy reactions than headaches, rashes, and hay fever. Allergies can cripple a victim. Nutrition's role in aiding the allergic is dramatic. (See chapter eight.)

It hastens convalescence.

Unrelieved stress, disease, lack of exercise, surgery, poor eating habits—all quickly rob the body of nutrients which must be replaced. Shorten these periods of anguish through proper eating habits. (See chapter 11.)

It fosters family love.

Nutrition's role in keeping marriages happy may be more significant than imagined. Homemakers who avoid "instant" foods and concentrate on developing culinary expertise will fortify themselves against boredom in the home. In addition, they will make fewer trips to doctors of medicine and psychiatry.

Nothing in your life is unaffected by nutrition. Without it you can't think; without it you can't work; without it you can't play; without it you can't love God, your neighbor, or yourself.

CHAPTER TWO

Nutrition and Mental Stability

It may be that there are other undreamed-of possibilities of therapy.
But for the moment, we have nothing better at our disposal than
the technique of psychoanalysis.... I am firmly convinced that one
day all of these disturbances we are trying to understand will be
treated by means of hormones or similar substances.

—Sigmund Freud,
Father of modern psychoanalysis
Autobiographical writings (1927)

Unlike psychotherapy, the science of nutrition is based on the exact science of biochemistry. When a person seeks help from psychotherapy, the therapist attempts to find the problem by interpreting what the patient tells him. Psychotherapy assumes that the mental or emotional oppression is the result of unresolved conflicts and then proceeds to treat the ailment according to the therapist's particular persuasion.

A psychologist aligned with the Freudian viewpoint might interpret a patient's complaints as unconscious conflicts resulting from repressed sexual desires remembered from childhood. A therapist with the viewpoint of Carl Jung would probably take a different line of strategy. Both techniques would require long-term counseling sessions. Therapists or analysts who are disciples of Otto Rank or Erich Fromm or Carl Rogers will all approach a patient's case differently.

The nutritionist attempts to rescue a patient from psychological difficulty by altering the physiological processes that are causing it. Numerous case histories are recorded which demonstrate the dramatic benefits of nutrition. Every patient needing relief from mental instability should at least try the nutritional route. It can't possibly hurt, and there is much to be gained.

"It has long been known that a deficiency of a single vitamin, nicotinic acid, can cause psychosis," says George Watson, Ph.D., in his book *Nutrition and Your Mind.* "This illness," Dr. Watson adds, "can be cured by administering niacin or its amide. Other vitamins in addition to niacin also have been implicated in the etiology of specific mental disorders."[1]

Pantothenic acid (a member of the B-complex vitamins) played an important role in the case of a young Ph.D. dropout whom medical researcher George Watson met quite by accident at a party in Los Angeles.

Bob had earned high marks as an undergraduate and had finished the first year of his studies toward a doctor's degree in mathematics when the U.S. Army drafted him.

In college his mind had been active and ambitious. After the Armed Forces experience he was without goals and lethargic. Dr. Watson suggested Bob be tested to determine whether his altered personality was due to a chemical imbalance.

"My brother's a doctor," Bob replied. "He tells me I'm physically 100 percent."

Dr. Watson, surprised by the remark, indicated that medicine didn't yet have such categorical answers and persuaded Bob to submit to the tests. They revealed that Bob was a low oxidizer, not burning food fast enough to draw sufficient energy from what he ate. Before entering the service he had been characterized as an achiever through a high level of brain and nervous system activity. Now it was discovered that his energy output was about 25 percent below average.

Supplements of pantothenic acid were prescribed in the form of calcium pantothenate tablets to be taken after breakfast. Five months later he was a different man. He reapplied for admission to his former university graduate school. Two years later he was awarded the Ph.D. degree in mathematics. Because Bob's brother had told him supplemental vitamins were "simply high-priced placebos," Bob nearly missed the simple nutritional rescue that changed his life.

Another entry in Dr. Watson's files illustrates again how the mind and emotions are affected by the body's modulating metabolism.

An attorney and his wife were on the brink of separation, and neither knew quite why they had let themselves become so incompatible. Following a vacation trip to Central America they were visiting casually one evening when the wife suddenly lost her temper, grabbed her husband's golf trophy, and slammed it through the front window.

The husband was terrified by the sound of shattering glass and by the sudden demonstration of his wife's fury. He was even more perplexed when she ran from the room screaming and sobbing, grabbed her coat, and left in the family car.

"I just sat," the attorney related. "I was scared."

His wife returned shortly afterward, went to bed, and

stayed there for the entire night and most of the following day. When she awakened she did not recall what she had done.

Tests later revealed a simple nutritional explanation for the nightmare. The couple had left on their trip happy as larks. To spare themselves the discomfort of diarrhea in a strange country they had taken heavy doses of sulfa drugs. After returning home, the wife continued to take small doses, avoiding carbohydrates to take off a few added pounds.

The sulfa drugs had rid their bowels of both the unfriendly bacteria and the normal "healthy" bacterial population (intestinal flora) as well.

"The flora synthesize a number of vitamins such as riboflavin, biotin, and vitamin K—of great importance to the energy-producing activities of the tissues, particularly the nervous system," Dr. Watson explained. "We have observed many abnormal psychological reactions in patients whose intestinal flora had been suppressed by drugs, or for any other reason, such as incorrect diet. These abnormal reactions include depression, anxiety, social withdrawal, irritability and excitability—and a tendency to lose self-control."

A corrected diet restored the couple to their former emotional stability.

In high school, Rod Snook of Whittier, California, was outgoing and intensely competitive in sports. His grades were high and his future looked bright. Rod made the principal's honor roll and the All-League First Team basketball squad. He was on the All Orange County Third Team and started with the Orange County All-Star game.

"On the exterior, I seemed to be aggressive and high strung," Rod told us. "But in reality, an illness was slowly driving me into a painful depression."

Following high school graduation Rod enrolled at
Orange Coast College in the fall of 1972. Physically and
mentally he alternated between hyperactivity and extreme
fatigue followed by depression. Despite his illness, Rod
pushed ahead as All-League on the college's second
basketball team, and became second leading scorer and
rebounder. He pushed himself "due to peer pressure and
the fact that I was learning basketball techniques and fun-
damentals from a great coach."

Slowly Rod began to lose his battle. "I had no control of
my illness because it was biochemical," he said. "But I was
unable to say no to the increasing demands of the game."

A variety of physicians and psychologists offered counsel, trying to control Rod's increasingly wide mood swings.
He was forced to turn down attractive scholarships to colleges throughout the United States because of the en-
croaching illness which remained a mystery.

Severe depression became his constant companion. One
afternoon he could stand the tension no longer. Rod locked
himself in the garage, took forty-eight sleeping pills,
climbed into his car, and started the engine.

Approximately thirty-five minutes later a woman mail
carrier noticed the closed door and heard the car's engine.
She phoned the paramedics who rushed the suicidal victim
to a nearby hospital. The quick work of friends spared the
young man's life.

The turning point in his downward spiral was provided
by a medical doctor trained also as a psychologist.
Megavitamin therapy coupled with electric convulsive
therapy (shock treatments) gave dramatic relief.

"After the fifth treatment I was sleeping for the first
time in six years," Rod recalls. "It was a true, deep sleep
without constant mind-wandering and restlessness. The
Lord saved me. I was completely a changed person."

Megavitamin therapy is an orthomolecular approach to

curing biochemical imbalances, Rod explained, adding confidentially: "The Lord was watching over me. There was a reason for the illness."

Rod's most critical stage was reached in the summer, peaking in October. The future had looked dark. Physicians diagnosed his illness as pancreatitis—an acute inflammation and blockage of the pancreatic duct. They likened the effects of Rod's chemical imbalance to a mild L.S.D. trip.

"The doctors said the stressful ordeal I had been going through for four years had caused the organ to fail. The pancreatitis placed me in a coma. Doctors said an operation would cause the pancreas to hemorrhage, leading to my death. For twenty-four hours I lay unconscious awaiting God's will. Finally the pancreatic duct opened. I was given a second chance."

Today Rod is a vital, enthusiastic young man. His weight has returned to 205 pounds. He joined the basketball squad of Biola College and later played for Whittier College with goals "disciplined by the strength of Jesus Christ."

"I want to give my athletic abilities to the Lord for a missionary trip with Overseas Crusades," Rod says. "I'm looking forward to improving my total life for Christ in the future."

Hitching the horse before the cart

Traditionally, physical and emotional illnesses have been treated with drugs and psychotherapy. Patients did not seek help until disease of body and mind had become clearly evident. That's changing rapidly. Biochemists are discovering preventive means through nutrition therapy which does much more than build and repair the body. The interplay of nutrients digested in the body may lead in a remarkable way to mental and emotional stability as well.

Speaking of the vast and exciting possibilities of healing mental disorders through nutrition, Henry Maudsley, the pioneering British psychiatrist, nearly a century ago complained of the disregard of physical factors in approaching mental disorders. He saw in medical doctors a deliberate resistance to recognition of the value of such treatment.

Said Maudsley in the nineteenth century: "The observations and classifications of mental disorders have been so exclusively psychological that we have not realized the fact that they illustrate the same pathological principles as other diseases, are produced the same way, and must be investigated in the same spirit of positive research. Until this is done, I see no hope of improvements in our knowledge of them and no use in multiplying books about them."

Oddly enough, Sigmund Freud agreed with Maudsley. Freud, often called the father of psychoanalysis, always insisted that patients seeking help for mental disorders should first be examined for physical disorders. But this basic premise was somehow forgotten in the enthusiastic reception of his new ideas on the subconscious. Psychiatry went on to highly developed forms, but very little was done to explore the possibilities of treating mental illness through nutrition.

The ninth estate

Widespread ignorance still prevails concerning the role of nutrition in psychological disorders a century after Maudsley criticized his colleagues. As it was in his day, so it is today: psychiatrists generally are trained to treat existing illnesses with drugs or psychotherapy. But many doctors are restless for another dimension to their work—the ninth factor in diagnosis—nutritional prevention and therapy. (The other eight considerations are the traditional factors of age, sex, occupation, residence, past history, family history, heredity, and stress.)

It is the view of Alan H. Nittler, a medical doctor in Santa Cruz, California, that many of his associates know they are doing less than their best. Wishing to strike out boldly, they are often afraid of such reprisals as a loss of license or a lack of patients, and the subsequent financial risks.

Yet Dr. Nittler sees a solution: the mastering of nutrition therapy and its relation to health and practice. He doesn't see the advancement of this viewpoint taking place yet in the sacrosanct halls of organized medicine. A paucity of curricula on nutrition exists in contemporary medical schools, although, thankfully, the winds seem to be changing.

Citizens of modern society, and the physicians who attend them, too often prefer to swallow pills to rid themselves of symptoms rather than to search for the cause of the pain. The pharmaceutical industry has made available every imaginable kind of medication to relieve the accompanying painful symptoms of disease. But every drug has a side effect, and can produce a contraindication for the patient which the doctor or research laboratory may discover too late.

How many nervous breakdowns, divorces, business failures, and dashed careers blamed on neuroses or psychoses might have been traced to purely physical causes and remedied by diet and sensible living habits?

Sweet tooth, sour disposition

The last organ of the body to be considered in most diets is the most important one of all—the brain. The mind can "burn" only sugar as fuel for thinking and for body control. Well then, why not eat sugar and plenty of it? There's a good reason why you should not.

The typical American starts his day with a breakfast of fruit juice, cereal, hotcakes, waffles, coffee cake, or toast. These are rapidly changed into sugar during digestion. In addition, refined sugar is usually sprinkled generously on the food or added by the manufacturers.

Within a few minutes after eating, this vast quantity of sugar hits the bloodstream. The blood sugar level can jump from 80 to 155 milligrams in minutes. The action calls out to the pancreas to produce insulin. "More! More!" cries the blood. The insulin allows the liver and muscles to withdraw sugar and store it as starch or glycogen or to change it into fat. This action prevents the sugar from being lost in the urine.

The body needs a controlled level of sugar in the blood to provide even amounts of energy. A flood of sugar overstimulates the pancreas, which overstimulates the liver, which draws from the blood too much sugar. Ironically, the result is fatigue.

Low blood sugar affects not only muscle energy but brain control as well. The area of the mind most quickly and seriously affected is the thalamic (emotional) area. Here lie the controls for regulating heartbeat, breathing, digestion, and many other functions. Here also lies the center for emotional control. Therefore a person whose blood sugar drops low begins to act and think like a neurotic or a psychotic. He develops fears and anxieties that are unjustified. He experiences gnawing fatigue, or claustrophobia, or depression serious enough to be suicidal.

Hyperinsulinism (commonly called "hypoglycemia") is an increasing malady which physicians are observing and charting. C. L. Derrick states in the *Oxford Looseleaf Medicine* periodical that "when seen for the first time and in the absence of a good history, the attack [of low blood sugar] may suggest some brain disease, such as infection, neoplasm [tumor] or vascular accident [apoplexy]. Because of their paroxysmal nature, the attacks may suggest epilepsy, acute alcoholism, amnesia, or some functional disorder such as hysteria. It is for these reasons that patients with hypoglycemia frequently are referred to neurological or psychiatric clinics."[2]

Biochemistry has also registered gains against the frightening disease of schizophrenia. Nobel-Prize-winning chemist Linus Pauling and David Hawkins found in their research that 94 percent of schizophrenic patients tested were deficient in ascorbic acid (vitamin C), pyridoxine (vitamin B_6), and niacinamide (vitamin B_3).

"A complete understanding of vitamins in relation to schizophrenia has not yet been obtained," they say. "There is uncertainty as to the relative contributions of genetic and environmental factors and to the effect of the schizophrenic episodes and of hospitalization on the biochemical and physiological functioning of the patients."

The researchers agreed, however, that "there is no uncertainty ... about the fact that the great majority, 94 percent, of the hospitalized schizophrenic subjects studied by us show a low urinary excretion of one or more of the three vitamins which we have studied, and that this is an indication of a low content of vitamins in the body, which can be rectified by the methods of orthomolecular psychiatry— the increased daily intake of the vitamins...."[3]

Pauling and Hawkins reminded readers that these vitamins are inexpensive and practically nontoxic—free of undesirable side reactions, as contrasted with ordinary drugs.

The next time you hear, "There's nothing physically wrong with you, go see a psychiatrist," take note. The aches, pains, depression, and mental instability might mean that your body needs the fine tuning of biochemistry instead of the couch.

Next year you will be the same person you are today, except for the friends you make, the books you read, and the food you eat.

THINGS TO DO

1. In cases of mental instability, always analyze the person's diet to see if an overconsumption of sugar is robbing the brain and the nervous system. Consult a nutritionist or an endocrinologist.

2. Do not rely solely on doctors of medicine to counsel you on doctrines of nutrition.

3. Avoid fad diets that totally eliminate carbohydrates. The body needs carbohydrates to convert the compounds into glucose to fuel the brain.

4. Supplement your diet with abundant amounts of vitamin B_1 (thiamine), B_6 (pyridoxine group), B_{12} (cobalamin group), niacin, pantothenic acid, and vitamin C.

5. Enjoy the good food in our varied recipes that follow. (See page 114 for chart on B vitamins and page 117 for chart on C vitamins.)

Queso (dip)

1 lb. Kraft Old English cheese

3 cups diced tomatoes with juice

2 cloves garlic through press

1 Tbsp. Worcestershire sauce

2 4-oz. cans Ortega green chiles, chopped

Place all the ingredients in a saucepan over low heat and stir until cheese is completely melted. When hot, transfer into a chafing dish and serve with tortilla chips.

Spanish Lady Guacamole

2 large ripe avocados
2 Tbsp. lime or lemon
  juice
2 tsp. olive oil
1 tsp. salt

¼ cup minced onion
4-oz. can Ortega diced
  green chiles
1 small tomato, diced

Puree avocados in blender. (Or mash well with a fork.) Add lime juice, olive oil, salt, onion, chiles, and diced tomato. Mix thoroughly and chill covered. Serve with corn chips or your own tortillas, cut and made crisp in hot oil. Remember, the wonderful avocado does darken, so plan to use it all—it doesn't store well.

Oriental Rumaki

⅓ cup soy sauce
½ cup maple syrup
2 Tbsp. cider vinegar
½ tsp. salt

12 chicken livers
18 bacon slices, cut in half
2 5-oz. cans water
  chestnuts

Mix liquids and salt together and set aside for marinade. Cut each liver into 3 or 4 pieces. Slice chestnuts in half and then into fourths. If chestnut is slim, slice into thirds. Place the liver and chestnut onto the slice of bacon. Wrap carefully and secure with a wooden toothpick. (Don't use plastic—they'll melt while baking.) Place appetizers in marinade, cover, and refrigerate several hours or overnight. Drain. Place on rack, set over a cookie sheet to catch the drippings, and bake in hot oven 400° about 20 minutes or until bacon is crisp. If necessary crisp the bacon at the last under the broiler. Drain on paper towels. Serves 36.

San Clemente Tuna Casserole*

8 oz. noodles (spinach
  noodles may be used)
¼ cup butter
½ cup chopped green
  onions
¼ cup chopped green
  pepper
¼ cup chopped celery
⅓ cup sifted flour (such
  as rice flour)
1 tsp. salt
2½ cups chicken broth
  (you may use bouillon)
½ cup white wine
½ cup heavy cream
½ to 1 cup fresh
  mushrooms
2 6-7-oz. cans tuna,
  drained
2 Tbsp. melted butter
1½ cups soft bread crumbs
¼ cup shredded cheddar
  cheese

In medium size saucepan melt butter and saute onions, pepper, and celery. Cook until tender. Blend in flour and salt and slowly stir in broth. Cook, stirring until sauce simmers and thickens. Add wine, cream, mushrooms, and tuna. Combine with noodles and turn into a greased casserole dish. Bake in 375° oven for 25 minutes. Remove from oven. Garnish with tomato wedges.

    Mix bread crumbs in butter and stir in cheese. Sprinkle on top and return to oven for 10 minutes. Remove from oven and allow to stand for 5-10 minutes before serving.

Courtesy Mrs. Manya Slevcove in San Clemente, Calif.

Stir-and-Pat Pastry

1 cup whole-wheat flour
1 cup unbleached flour
1 tsp. salt
½ cup safflower oil (or
  other vegetable oil with
  no cholesterol)

¼ cup cold nonfat milk or
  water

Measure flour and salt into sifter. Sift into bowl. Measure oil into one cup and add the measured milk. Pour all at once over the flour and stir with fork. Pat mixture together to form a ball. Divide in half for two crusts. Pat dough into 8″ or 9″ pan. Prick pastry and bake in hot 425° oven for 7-10 minutes. Cool before filling. Fill with the quiche recipe on page 41 or bake and serve with fruit, pie filling or ice cream.

Gems from the Seas

1 lb. fresh scallops
3 Tbsp. butter
1 Tbsp. chives
½ cup heavy cream

2 egg yolks, beaten
1 Tbsp. melted butter
¾ cup grated (Monterey)
  Jack cheese

Cut scallops in half. Sauté gently in butter and chives. Add cream and cook over medium heat 2-3 minutes. Remove scallops to a small flat casserole. Blend egg yolks and butter together and pour over scallops. Top with grated cheese. Bake until cheese is melted. Serve immediately. We reserve this expensive dish for a special treat. If you like, buy fewer scallops and use a more economical fish like turbot with it. It's mildly flavored and will blend nicely. Cut into chunks about the size of scallops.

Crabmeat Quiche

6½ oz. crabmeat, flaked
3 oz. Swiss cheese
3 oz. Gruyère cheese
8″ unbaked piecrust
2 eggs, slightly beaten

1 cup cream
1 Tbsp. flour
¼ tsp. salt
dash of cayenne pepper

Blend together well the crabmeat and cheeses. Distribute evenly over the piecrust. Mix beaten eggs, cream, flour, and seasonings. Pour over crab and cheese and pop into a hot oven 450° for 10 minutes. Lower temperature to 350° and bake for approximately one hour. Watch closely. Serve in small wedges as an appetizer.

CHAPTER THREE

Hope for the Hypoglycemic

Certain bodily maladies are fruitful foundations of despondency.
—Charles H. Spurgeon,
Nineteenth-century British evangelist

Charlie Brown, hero of the Peanuts comic strip, once sought the advice of his "psychiatrist" (Lucy in her booth). He poured out a long string of personal anguish and ended with a sigh of despair. When he was finished, Lucy stuck out her palm and said, "Your blood sugar is low. Five cents, please."

Lucy's diagnosis might have eased Charlie Brown's tensions for a while, but unless he did something about that metabolic upset he was probably back at the booth the following day, more depressed than ever.

"All emotions have biochemical as well as psychological elements," says Abraham Hoffer, M.D., Director of Psychiatric Research in Saskatchewan's Department of Public Health.[1]

Dr. Richard Horace Hoffmann believes that "most neuro-

43

tics are the way they are because some underlying and undiscovered bodily ailment contributes to their anxiety."[2]

For five cents, Charlie Brown had made this important discovery—that the metabolism of the body directly affects the emotions. Until Charlie Brown tunes up his anatomy, no amount of psychological counseling will totally eliminate his doldrums.

From moods to foods

Increasing numbers of Americans are suffering the crazy-quilt pattern of painful and puzzling physical symptoms from the shock waves of abnormal plunges in blood sugar levels. Why? Because statistics today show that for one person in every ten, sugar can be a deadly ingredient.

It is a curious fact that many physicians today do not recognize hypoglycemia as a valid medical problem. Yet in 1949 Dr. Seale Harris of Birmingham, Alabama, was honored by the American Medical Association for conducting research which led to the discovery of hypoglycemia. The AMA gave Dr. Harris its Distinguished Service Medal after he observed that some patients who were not diabetic and who had not been treated with insulin still went into "insulin shock."

This condition is just the opposite of diabetes. In most cases of hypoglycemia, the pancreas is overactive, producing too much insulin. So the effect can be similar to the reaction of a diabetic when he takes an overdose of insulin: shock, dizziness, irritability, cold sweats, shakiness, nervousness, anxiety—possibly even collapse.

"A piece of candy or a glass of orange juice (13 percent sugar) will rescue the diabetic from insulin shock. Will it help the person with an overactive pancreas? No—for a very simple reason," say the authors of *Low Blood Sugar and You*. "The pancreas works because sugar has been eaten. (If it didn't, you'd be diabetic.) If the pancreas is overactive, sugar isn't going to quiet it down; it will stimulate the gland still more."[3] So the hypoglycemic person will make himself worse in the long run if he eats sugar.

However, this does not really explain the disorder called hypoglycemia. The malfunction of the pancreas is really itself only a symptom whose true origin can only be guessed at. Yet our best evidence indicates that an overconsumption of sugar (which most Americans are guilty of) is the culprit.

It is interesting to note that in 1973 the American Medical Association capriciously labeled hypoglycemia a "non-disease." Despite the award to Dr. Harris in 1949, and despite the fact that hypoglycemia has been shown to be the villain in many emotional and physical complaints, the AMA has legislated it out of its dictionary of diseases. This hasn't changed anything. Americans go on eating an average of 126 pounds of processed sugar per person per year and paying the price in poor health both for how they eat and what they eat.

The body requires a good nutritional boost to start the day, yet many Americans skip breakfast altogether. On top of that they load it with caffeine and sugar at a coffee break, punishing the body further. The empty calories of the sugar are a chemical threat to the body because they lack the B vitamins and minerals necessary for their assimilation. So the body must rob the vitamins from other foods or from the body's store, causing a B-complex and mineral deficiency which can lead to emotional upset.

You don't think you eat that much sugar? If all the food you buy in the supermarket were accurately labeled you would discover that 90 percent of your average purchases probably contained sugar. Approximately 19 percent of the average American's calorie source is sugar. The sugar content of some products inspected went as high as 68 percent. The hypoglycemic is in as much danger as the diabetic because the Food and Drug Administration does not demand complete disclosure of all diluents, binders, fillers, flavoring agents, and sweeteners.

Perhaps the worst outrage is the damage such food does to babies and children. Our family doctor feels strongly that a contributing factor to juvenile delinquency today is sugar-saturated food.

Grading health on the curve

To determine whether you have hypoglycemia, you must take the five- or six-hour glucose tolerance test in a laboratory, administered by a doctor. The purpose of this test is to determine the dynamics of your body's handling of sugar over a period of time. After you drink a glucose-laden, carbonated liquid, a blood sample is taken every hour and a chart prepared. At the end of the test the chart indicates the manner in which the body metabolizes its sugar. Normally, after consumption of sugar, the blood level will rise until insulin is produced; then it will gradually fall to a "fasting" level. But in the person with hypoglycemia, the sugar level will drop significantly at some point or points during the glucose tolerance test rather than maintaining a normal fasting level. In extreme cases of hypoglycemia, even after taking sugar a patient may find he has less sugar in his blood than when the test began. That is why sufferers often crave sugar. To succumb to a quick-energy sugar intake may temporarily alleviate the symptoms, but will ultimately make the condition worsen.

The person who wishes to pursue the diagnosis and cure of hypoglycemia should be prepared for a measure of resistance and confusion by some medical doctors. The American Medical Association is on record as calling the disease a myth. Physicians have reasons for criticizing some "sugar doctors" who broadcast this oversimplified diagnosis.

"Hypoglycemia is not a disease," Sydney Walker III wrote in the July 1975 issue of *Psychology Today*. "It is a physiological state that can occur for various reasons."

Walker underscores the sophistication of the bodily functions which convert carbohydrates into glucose, and glucose into energy and fuel for the nervous system. This process involves the liver, the adrenal glands, the pituitary and thyroid glands, the pancreas, and often the endocrine glands. Trouble anywhere along the line can lead to low blood sugar levels (hypoglycemia) or to sugar levels that are too high (diabetes). A tumor on the pancreas, for example, could cause overstimulation of that vital organ. Other defects in metabolism that are congenital or the result of disease can be the culprits. Thus hypoglycemia itself is not a disease but a symptom indicative of a metabolic problem. Specific diagnosis and treatment of the glands affected in each individual case must be the rule.

But on one point there is no argument: Refined white sugar is in no way beneficial to our bodies. You do not need to eat sugar or excessive concentrated starches which the body turns to sugar. We'll go one step beyond: You'll do your teeth, your heart, your arteries, your pancreas, and your nervous system a favor by cutting out these empty calories for good. Don't let advertising lures convince you that sugar is necessary for energy and well being. It is not.

Sugar drunks

Look around. Victims of Big C (for "carbohydrates") abound.

Our friend Sally Hanson (not her real name) was one. A spirited person through her childhood, Sally entered married life with optimism and abundant energy.

Several years later Sally noticed a general slowdown in her physical makeup. Getting out of bed became a drag. She developed headaches, heart palpitations, and general feelings of exhaustion. Her doctor gave her numerous blood tests, EKGs, and other sophisticated examinations, but the specter of fatigue continued to haunt her. The doctor then prescribed tranquilizers; later he ordered ten aspirin tablets a day; still later, tranquilizers were again prescribed and more tests in a fruitless crusade to find Sally's trouble.

The family dentist provided the turning point in Sally's miserable life by giving her a book to read. "That's me!" Sally found herself exclaiming continually as she read *Body, Mind & Sugar,* by E. M. Abrahamson, M.D., and A. W. Pezet. "That's my situation exactly." When she had finished the book Sally phoned her doctor and asked for the six-hour glucose tolerance test suggested by the book.

"Why?" he asked.

"I think I might be hypoglycemic," she replied.

"It's a fad these days to be 'hypoglycemic,' " the doctor told her. "You don't really need that test. The reason people—especially women—think they're hypoglycemic is because they get out of bed in the morning, have a roll and coffee for breakfast, play tennis until noon, have a martini and a weight-watcher lunch, and then expect their bodies to function normally."

The physician was right in his view of the all-too-common American eating habits. But experience shows that such dietary abuse over a long period does indeed result in the exhaustion of the adrenal glands and problems with an overworked pancreas. This is what changed Sally from a vivacious wife and mother into a bedridden complainer.

The doctor reluctantly arranged for the six-hour glucose tolerance test as his patient requested, and her graph was charted. It ended with an alarming blood sugar level of only 22 points (22 milligrams percent or 22 milligrams per 100 cc. of blood). The initial blood sugar level should lie between 80 and 120 mg. per 100 cc. of blood. The level should rise to not more than 160 in 30 or 60 minutes, and it should return to its initial value within two hours.

"There's been a mistake," her physician decided as he studied Sally's chart. "You'd be dead if your level actually dropped that low."

"Well, that's what I've been feeling like for the past two years," Sally declared.

"I can't believe this is correct. I'll schedule you for another series—this time at the hospital. I want to see the results of another lab."

But the second chart read exactly the same. The physician prescribed a high-protein diet with no sugar, and within a month Sally began to feel good. Gradually she returned to rosy health. She eliminated from her diet caffeine, an abundance of carbohydrates, and refined sugar. Because the new diet made such a difference in her life, Sally won't cheat.

"Our bodies are like a three-legged stool," she told us. "They function best with a proper balance of food, rest, and exercise."

Fifteen years and $25,000

A schoolteacher in her late twenties told us she had spent approximately half her life and some $25,000 pursuing an elusive cure for chronic ill health before discovering she was hypoglycemic.

During her last year at UCLA she began feeling unusually tired at the end of her walk from classroom to car for the trip home. More and more, fatigue plagued her, requiring increased hours of sleep, until she was forced to drop several classes in order to make it through the year.

She spent the summer resting at the beach before entering her first year as a high school teacher. When she spoke about her troubles to physicians they said they could find nothing wrong, and told her it must be her "nerves." No doctor mentioned diet or quizzed her on what she was eating.

"Overwork" was a frequent conclusion from the medical community. One doctor suggested she keep candy in her purse to eat regularly through the day. She heard the diagnosis "neurasthenia" (fatigue of the nerves) applied to her condition and she submitted to lengthy and expensive treatments at a San Diego clinic. She received not a glimmer of hope. She was told that her body had been born tired, and that fatigue was something she would have to live with for the rest of her life.

Following her first glucose tolerance test, some clues to the causes of her ill health began to emerge. She was put on a high-protein diet, modified with some fruit sugar and carbohydrates to accommodate a sluggish liver. The teacher has been rewarded by slow but definite traces of strength returning to her body.

"Today I'm fine if I watch my diet," she said. Now a counselor in private practice, she told us: "I still tend to overdo, but that's my fault and I can control my schedule."

A glucose tolerance test a decade and a half earlier would have spared her the expense, depression, and fatigue which plagued her for years.

Coked up and blacked out

A husky high school athlete in Escondido, California, became addicted to cokes during his early teen years. At the age of seventeen the young man could no longer outrun the onslaught of that much sugar.

Often after a game of tennis he would lose consciousness. Sometimes he would drive to the opposite side of town in a dazed condition to visit his girl friend.

"I would open the door and find Dick standing there without seeing me," Lory recalls. "I would help him inside and run quickly to get some orange juice. Then I'd wait for approximately fifteen minutes until his consciousness returned."

Dick grew worse, eventually having barely enough energy to drag himself to the breakfast table where his mother served heaping portions of pancakes, French toast, and other foods loaded with carbohydrates.

An alert doctor arranged for a glucose tolerance test which revealed Dick's true condition: a severe case of hypoglycemia. Now with a sugarless diet that offers plentiful supplies of protein, Dick's blackouts have ceased. So have his intense periods of anger and anxiety.

Spaced-out on sweets

The parents of a sixth-grade boy noticed a gradual deterioration of their son's mental attitude and physical condition. At night Scott began to hallucinate, complaining that "someone has me by the throat."

In school he became listless and unchallenged by sports or studies. His worried parents arranged for comprehensive physical examinations, but there seemed to be nothing wrong. The doctor prescribed sleeping pills which worked for a short time. Scott's hands trembled in school. He couldn't compete in sports. Depression hounded him, and his report card showed a downward spiral of failing grades.

A casual phone call from a friend was the start of Scott's healing. His mother and father arranged an interview with Mrs. Gladys Lindberg, head of Lindberg Nutrition Centers throughout southern California. As soon as Mrs. Lindberg saw Scott she said, "This child is on sleeping pills. If you don't get him off those he'll be in a mental institution before he's fifteen years old!"

After a glucose tolerance test showed his blood sugar to be low, Scott faithfully followed the Lindberg diet: no sugar, high protein, and vitamin-mineral food supplements. He began to respond immediately.

Today Scott is normal, happy, and in step with good nutrition. He knows what he can and cannot eat to feel good and accomplish the most. Save for the sound guidance his parents received, he could just as easily be headed for a mental institution and a wasted life.

The late show

A graduate in cinematography from USC became so skilled in her profession that she was in demand for presentations in many parts of the country. One night, after noting a puzzling decline in strength, the young woman fell unconscious on the floor of her office and had to be revived by friends.

After that frightful experience, to acquire enough energy to lecture she began taking malted milk shakes with her to provide an energy kick. But she discovered that the sweet "high" didn't last. Instead, it plunged her energy level lower as her blood sugar dropped and exhaustion returned.

Not until she nearly gave up her career was she rescued by a nutritionist. Today she adheres strictly to a prescribed high-protein diet without sugar. This simple combination has restored her health, her job, and her enthusiasm for life.

We wonder: Does the average medical doctor know how poorly his patients eat? Probably not. If he did, wouldn't he turn from casual attitudes about nutrition to a more crusading stance?

If you still sing, as Mary Poppins did, that a spoonful of sugar makes the medicine go down, you should remember what happens to your constitution when those empty calories hit the bloodstream. Chances are good that you'll avoid both sugar and medicine in favor of body-building nutrition over the long, consistent haul.

Have midmorning and midafternoon snacks of cheese, milk, nuts, and fruit for long-lasting energy. You don't need to give up desserts. Just eat delectables made tasty by natural, nutritious sweeteners.

THINGS TO DO

1. Avoid all foods containing refined, white sugar as much as possible.

2. Extreme fatigue, mental depression, emotional upsets, nervousness, and a craving for sweets or alcohol can be early signs of hypoglycemia. If you or anyone in your family is not functioning at peak level and has these symptoms, seek the help of an endocrinologist or a medical doctor who has a nutritional approach to the healing arts.

3. Hypoglycemia is a forerunner of diabetes. Discover it early.

4. If necessary, observe the anti-hypoglycemia diet, under the direction of a physician. Don't try to treat yourself exclusively. Relief is possible through specific diet alterations and specified vitamin and mineral supplements. Find a doctor who is especially interested in this disorder. If you do not experience progress within a reasonable amount of time, seek other medical help.

5. Enjoy the healthful, sugarless dessert recipes on pages 62 through 70.

Anti-Hypoglycemia Diet

Recommended by our medical doctor

Three rules to follow:
1. Eliminate all sugar.
2. Eat no refined carbohydrates.
3. Eat low amounts of fat.

Foods allowed:

Lean meat: Fowl (fat free), sea foods, if not packed in oil.

Dairy products: Certified raw nonfat milk (if available), whole milk if you are underweight; butter in small amounts; skim-milk cheese (such as cottage cheese, string cheese, or hoop cheese); yogurt and custards.

Eggs: Only one daily.

Whole fruit: An orange or a banana daily.

Raw nuts: Preferably dry roasted and nut butters, unless weight or cholesterol is a problem. Use nuts for snacks between meals.

Bread: Seven-grain or other whole wheat. Oat, soya, high gluten, sprouted grain bread. Seven-grain is preferred.

Cereal: Seven-grain to cook, or granola-type cereals.

Whole soybean products.

Artichoke or spinach macaroni and spaghetti. Use for casseroles.

Foods to avoid:

All sugars and refined carbohydrates.

Corn, rice, packaged cereals (whole-grain rice, whole-grain cereals permitted).

Canned fruit—especially sugar packed.

Pie, cake, pastries, candies.

Dates, raisins, and other dried fruit.
All cola drinks and sugar soft drinks.
Coffee and strong tea.
All alcoholic beverages.
All animal fats and especially cooked animal fats: no
  sausage, bacon, weiners, fatty sandwich meats, or
  hamburger (but *lean* ground round is OK).
No smoking. Definitely can cause hypoglycemia, as well
  as many other diseases.

Recommended breakfast:

Any whole fruit (preferable to the juice).
One egg or *lean* meat of any kind (if cholesterol high,
  eat fewer eggs).
Pat of butter (small)—some patients to have no but-
  ter.
One slice whole-wheat bread.
Milk or herb tea. Coffee (decaffeinated if you can't
  resist coffee).

10 A.M. morning snacks (choice of):

Milk or piece of fruit.
Gelatin (without sugar) mixed with fresh fruit or veg-
  etables.
Raw nuts (preferable to dry-roasted or processed).
Nut-mix (nuts, pumpkin seeds, sunflower seeds, and
  raisins, mixed one-fourth each.
Protein wafers or tablets (from health food stores).

Lunch:

Soup without starch.
Fresh fruit, fresh vegetable or fish salad.
Serving of lean meat, seafood or cheese.
Choice of vegetable.
Milk, buttermilk, or tomato juice.

Afternoon snack:

> Same as 10:00 A.M. snack.

Dinner:

> Soup without starch.
> Meat or seafood.
> Vegetables low in starch (lettuce, watercress, cucumbers, beet greens, radishes, etc.)
> Dressing: vinegar and oil or blue cheese.
> Milk and/or herb tea.
> Fresh fruit.

Bedtime:

> Cheese and one glass of milk.

During the night:

> When awakened and cannot go back to sleep choose one of the following:
>> Glass of milk or unsweetened orange juice.
>> Cheese of any kind.
>> Sandwich made of whole-grain bread with cheese.
>> Nuts of any kind (preferably raw).
>> Protein wafers or tablets.
>> Protein milk drink.

Nutritional supplement:

> A multi-vitamin/mineral tablet morning and evening.
> Additional 1,000 mg. of vitamin C.
> Safflower oil capsule morning and night.

Coffee—A Drug on the Market

Americans brew approximately 2½ billion pounds of coffee annually, and are not the better for it. Heavy coffee drinkers who miss their morning coffee can experience a variety of feelings resembling withdrawal symptoms from drugs: irritability, headache, inefficient work, nervousness, restlessness, and (surprisingly) lethargy.

Caffeine speeds up the heart and interferes with digestion. In addition to caffeine there are numerous substances in the roasted bean, including carbohydrates (sucrose, pectins, starch, hemicellulose, and lignin), oils, protein, ash, and acids (chlorogenic, caffeic, quinic, oxalic, malic, citric, and tartaric).

Scientists at the University of Wisconsin have produced multiple B-vitamin deficiencies merely by feeding animals coffee. It seems that caffeine, by stimulating the heartbeat, increases the flow of blood plasma through the kidneys and thus causes more of the B vitamins to be lost in the urine.

Excessive use of coffee, cigarettes, and alcohol is related to the level of blood sugar; they stimulate the production of adrenal hormones which cause the blood sugar to be increased, thus producing the desired boost. But the pancreas soon secretes insulin, causing the sugar level to fall again. Result: irritability from low blood sugar. It's often a factor in divorce, office feuds, and poor scholastic records.

Coffee does sometimes calm hyperkinetic children. And adults like it because it stimulates the mind, banishes drowsiness and fatigue, and leads to a more perfect association of ideas in the brain. But there is the piper to pay for this false lift.

Persons with known coronary disease should drink coffee moderately. Coffee drinkers, it has been shown, run greater risk of bladder cancer.

Decaffeinated coffee is not without sin. It stimulates gastric secretions to a limited extent because of other constituents of the bean. Individuals with peptic ulcers should consume their coffee (if at all) during meals, well diluted with cream.

The aroma of coffee is alluring; the taste is magnificent. But if health is your first concern, coffee is one luxury you might well do without.

Caffeine Content of Popular Drinks

One Cup:

Brewed Coffee	80 - 120 mg.
Instant Coffee	66 - 100 mg.
Decaffeinated Coffee	1 - 6 mg.
Leaf Tea	30 - 75 mg.
Bagged Tea	42 - 100 mg.
Instant Tea	30 - 60 mg.
Cocoa	up to 50 mg.
Cola Drinks	15 - 30 mg.

Caffeine levels in soft drinks can affect brain development in young children.

Sugar Is Sweet, and So?

Sugar is sweet and dangerous to your health. The tragic fact is that Americans eat more than one-sixth of all their calories in the form of visible sugar or sugar that has been added to prepared foods and drinks. This adds up to an astounding average of approximately two pounds per person per week!

A person can quite easily wind up a day believing he has had no sugar at all when actually he has one or two cups of it in processed food consumed. Sugar causes tooth decay; it overstimulates insulin flow and ruins appetites.

Blood sugar rises more rapidly when refined sugars are

eaten than when natural sweets are a part of the diet. Honey and fruit sugars provide high mineral and enzyme content; refined sugar has nothing but calories. Natural sweets are beneficial for food and energy and are kinder to the system than the shock treatment of processed sweets.

The difference between natural and refined sugar can be graphically illustrated by a simple test. Serve one hungry person a pound of dates and a second hungry person a pound of chocolates. Can you guess who will eat more? The date-eater will have a hard time finishing the pound because a bodily reflex causes the alimentary canal to gag on a surfeit of food; the candy eater probably will eat more of the pound. When refined sweets are a part of the diet, overeating is the natural consequence. But when natural sweets make up a diet, gluttony is rare.

Nothing's sweeter than honey

This healthful substance not only comes from the busy bees, but also is distilled from trees as "vegetable honey" (often called "manna" by chemists).

A natural product, honey is high in mineral content and tastes nearly twice as sweet as sugar. Adults and infants tolerate honey equally well. Because honey contains such a high percentage of minerals, it does not decay the teeth like processed sugar.

The sugar in honey—fructose—is much easier for the body to assimilate. A lesser amount of insulin is needed to metabolize fructose than is needed for sucrose (which is basically all other sugars). Honey is rich in copper which helps to assimilate iron.

> Kind words are like honey—
> enjoyable and healthful.
> —Proverbs 16:24 *The Living Bible*

Dr. Currier's Breakfast Cocktail

1 or 2 glasses of whole (*certified* only) raw milk (if available)

1 or 2 eggs

1 or 2 Tbsp. powdered milk

1 Tbsp. wheat germ or rice polishings

1 Tbsp. primary food yeast or brewer's yeast

1 Tbsp. lecithin granules

1 Tbsp. cold processed sesame seed oil, safflower oil, or wheat germ oil

1 Tbsp. powdered liver-protein (low heat, desiccated liver powder is an excellent source of protein and natural vitamins. However, if the taste of liver is objectionable, use a smaller amount; or chunks of beef liver may be frozen and grated into the cocktail.)

You may add any of the following for variety and sweetness: fresh orange, pineapple, banana, pure peanut butter, carob powder, honey, blackstrap molasses, powdered coconut, frozen unsweetened fruit juice, nutmeg, cinnamon, vanilla, dash of salt and yogurt (never add sugar).

Basic Eggnog

2-3 Tbsp. powdered milk

2 cups milk

2 eggs

1 Tbsp. honey

1 tsp. vanilla

1-2 Tbsp. brewer's yeast

2 ice cubes

Beat all ingredients together in blender. Serve immediately. Add for variations: banana, avocado, pear, peach, or apricot. For building strength, add more powdered milk and brewer's yeast.

High-Protein Milk

1 quart milk
3 cups dry milk
¼ cup malted milk powder
¼ cup soy powder
¼ cup honey

Blend all ingredients together and keep covered in the refrigerator. One cup of this nutritious drink provides 30 grams of protein. Use this for a quick energy boost instead of coffee.

Adapting Natural Sweeteners to Take the Place of Granulated Sugar

Honey

¾ cup = 1 cup sugar. Reduce liquid in recipe by one-fourth. (Or add ¼ cup flour or milk powder.) Reduce baking temperature by 25°. Most of the sweet recipes in this book call for the use of honey. It can be used in quick breads, cookies, snacks, cakes, ice cream, etc. You can also use honey for no-bake pies. Honey provides a delicious flavor with healthful benefits. Food prepared with honey will keep fresh and moist longer than food prepared with sugar.

Maple Syrup (Pure)

1½ cups = 1 cup sugar. Reduce liquid in recipe by one-half. This does not have the nutritional value of honey, and for those eliminating sugar this may not be allowed. However, this is much preferred to the sugar syrups that are generally used.

Molasses

1½ cups = 1 cup sugar. This makes cookies and cakes moist. Molasses is rich in minerals and other nutrients, making it an acceptable sweetener except for those on rigid diets.

These guidelines are not rigid. You should test and experiment so that your recipes will please your palate. These sweeteners do not offer the light texture that is characteristic of sugar, but the nutritional benefits are worth the aesthetic lack.

Home Cranked Vanilla Ice Cream

6 eggs, slightly beaten	2 cups honey
7 cups milk	½ tsp. salt
1 cup powdered milk	1 Tbsp. pure vanilla
3 cups whipping cream	

Beat eggs in large mixing bowl. Add remaining ingredients in the order given, blending well. Pour mixture into chilled freezing can and add the paddle. Stir in more milk if needed to bring mixture up to "full" line on the can. Follow manufacturer's freezing instructions.
Variation: If using fresh fruit, plan to add it about halfway through the freezing period.

Snack Mix

1 cup pecans, raw	1 cup raisins, moist
1 cup peanuts, salted	1 cup sunflower seeds, raw
1 cup cashews, raw	1 cup soy nuts, roasted
1 cup almonds, raw	1 cup pumpkin seeds, raw

Toss all together in a large bowl. We keep this snack in a cookie jar instead of cookies. When putting out a dish of this snack, add pitted prunes. However, don't add the prunes to the jar. The nuts absorb too much moisture from the prunes and lose their crispness.

Orange Cheese Pie Ala Peaches

Graham cracker crust:

1½ cups graham cracker crumbs (approximately 20 single crackers)

⅓ cup melted butter

Place graham crackers in a plastic bag and roll out until fine. Combine with butter and press into a 9″ pie plate.

Filling

12 oz. cream cheese

3 eggs

3 Tbsp. frozen orange juice concentrate from 6 oz. can.

½ cup honey

⅓ cup powdered milk

2 tsp. grated orange rind

Soften cheese to room temperature and beat until fluffy. Add eggs one at a time and continue beating. Then add juice, honey, and milk solids, combining well. Stir in orange rind with a spoon. Pour into pie shell and bake for 25 minutes in 350° oven, or until set. Remove and cool for 5 minutes. Then cover with topping.

Topping

1 cup dairy sour cream

1 Tbsp. orange juice concentrate

1 tsp. honey

1 tsp. vanilla

Stir all ingredients together and pour over cheese filling. Return to oven for 7 minutes. Remove and cool quickly. Refrigerate while preparing peaches.

Peach glaze

Remaining orange juice concentrate (approximately ½ cup)

2 tsp. cornstarch

4 peaches

Pour orange juice in saucepan and stir in corn starch. Cook slowly until thickened. Cool. Slice peaches and arrange on pie evenly and in the same direction. Spoon orange juice sauce over peaches and chill until serving time.

St. John's Fudge

½ cup sifted carob powder
1 Tbsp. safflower oil
3 Tbsp. butter, softened
½ cup peanut butter
⅓ cup honey
1 tsp. vanilla

¾ cup powdered milk
½ cup sunflower seeds,
  chopped fine in blender
½ cup pecans, crushed in
  plastic bag

Measure into mixing bowl the first six ingredients and stir well. Slowly add powdered milk and beat until smooth. Add seeds and nuts. Mixture will be heavy. Blend with a wooden spoon or your hands and press into a buttered 10″ × 6″ pan. Refrigerate until firm. Cut into squares. Makes 24 pieces. This can easily be doubled.

Milk-and-Honey Fudge

½ stick butter, softened to
  room temperature
½ cup honey
¼ cup soy powder (or soy
  flour)

1½ cups powdered milk
⅓ cup coarsely chopped
  pecans

Beat butter and honey together with a wooden spoon. Blend in soy powder. Add the dry milk in small amounts and beat until smooth. Mixture will be heavy. Add nuts and press into buttered 10″ × 6″ pan. Chill and cut into squares. This makes a delicious lunch treat.

Variations: Add grated orange rind or coconut. Use almonds, walnuts, or other nuts. Use fudge to stuff pitted dates.

Christmas Calico Fudge

½ cup pure peanut butter
2 Tbsp. peanut oil
2 Tbsp. honey
⅔ cup powdered milk
⅓ cup candied fruit (as in
  fruitcake mix)

1 cup nuts (½ almonds, ½
  pecans)
⅓ cup sesame seeds

Mix peanut butter, oil, and honey together. Add milk in small amounts and beat until smooth. Fold in fruit, nuts, and seeds. Press into a 9″ buttered pan. Refrigerate until firm. Cut into squares and serve. Store covered in refrigerator.

Variation: Candied pineapple and fresh dates in place of candied fruit.

Candied Fruit
(for fruitcakes)

1 cup honey
⅓ cup water
1 Tbsp. vanilla

Fruits:
  apple chunks
  cherries
  orange & lemon peel
  pineapple chunks

Mix honey and water in saucepan and bring to a boil. Add vanilla. Place the fresh fruit into the syrup and cook until tender, stirring often. Remove and drain. Allow to cool before using. This fruit may be prepared in the summer when cherries and pineapple are in season; then freeze until time to use in fruitcakes, cookies, or Calico Fudge at Christmastime.

Peanut Butter Cookies

1 cup peanut butter
1 cup honey
½ cup oil
2 Tbsp. butter
1 tsp. vanilla
1 cup powdered milk

1 cup rolled oats
1 cup whole-wheat pastry
   flour
¼ cup soy flour
1 tsp. salt
1 cup crushed peanuts

Mix peanut butter, honey, oil, butter, and vanilla together. Add dry milk and oats, stirring well. Measure flours and salt into sifter and sift gradually into peanut butter mixture and blend. Add crushed peanuts and form into walnut-size balls. Place on oiled cookie sheet and flatten with the tines of a fork. Bake in moderate 350° oven for 10 minutes or until lightly browned. Cool on rack before storing.

Carrot Cookies

¼ cup butter
¼ cup vegetable oil
½ cup honey
1 egg
¾ cup whole-wheat flour
¼ cup soy flour*
¼ tsp. salt
½ tsp. cinnamon
1 tsp. baking powder
½ cup raw bran

½ cup powdered nonfat
   milk
1 cup carrots, grated
   (nutmeg grater works
   well)
½ cup raisins
¼ cup sesame seeds or
   nuts
1 tsp. vanilla

Cream butter, oil, and honey. Add egg and beat. Measure flour, salt, cinnamon, and baking powder into sifter and sift into creamed mixture. Stir in remaining ingredients, blending well. Drop by teaspoons onto lightly oiled cookie sheet. Bake in 350° oven for 12-15 minutes.

*Whole-wheat flour may be substituted for soy.

Fresh Apricot Sherbet

2 tsp. lemon juice
½ cup evaporated milk
1 cup fresh apricots or
  canned in a water pack
1 cup unsweetened
  pineapple juice

3 Tbsp. honey (or artificial
  sweetener for diabetics)
1 envelope unflavored
  gelatin (1 Tbsp.)
¼ cup cold water

Blend lemon juice and milk together in small bowl. Place beaters in milk and chill in freezer until crystals form. Place apricots and juice in blender and whiz at high speed for several minutes. Slowly add 3 Tbsp. honey at high speed.

Soften gelatin in water and place over heat briefly to dissolve completely. Add to fruit mixture and then refrigerate until slightly thickened. Remove and beat until stiff. Whip the chilled milk and fold into the fruited gelatin. Spoon into sherbet dishes and garnish with fresh mint leaves. Keep cold until serving.

Vermont-Baked Apples

8 large Rome Beauty
  apples (or your favorite
  baking apple)

2-3 Tbsp. butter
1 cup *pure* Vermont maple
  syrup

Wash, core, and peel about ½″ down the apple. Place in glass baking dish. Dot each apple with about 1 tsp. butter in the core. Pour syrup over and into apples. Add a little hot water around the apples. Bake in preheated 350° oven for 1 hour or until tender. Baste with syrup during cooking. Serve warm or cold for breakfast or after-school snack. Delicious with topping of dairy sour cream or whipped cream with a dash of maple syrup.

Apple Crunch

½ stick butter
6 tart apples (Rome
   Beauty, McIntosh, or
   Jonathan)
1 tsp. cinnamon
3 tsp. sucaryl*

2 Tbsp. lemon juice (or
   orange juice)
1 cup granola (see recipe
   on page 251)
butter

Melt butter in 9″ cake pan. Pour off most of the butter into small bowl. Peel, core, and slice apples. Put into butter-coated pan. Sprinkle cinnamon over apples. Mix sweetener, juice, and remaining butter together and pour over apples. Spread granola evenly over fruit. Dot generously with additional butter. Bake for 40 minutes in 325° oven. Serve warm with half and half.

*The artificial sweetener is to accommodate the diabetic or severe hypoglycemic.

Honey-Baked Bananas

6 ripe bananas
2 Tbsp. butter
1 Tbsp. fresh lemon juice

¼ cup honey
¼ cup crushed peanuts

Peel bananas, cut in half and slice lengthwise. Place in shallow baking dish. Melt butter and combine with honey and lemon juice. Pour over bananas, coating well. Bake in slow oven at 325° for 15 minutes or until glazed. Garnish with nuts at serving. May be served warm or cold.
Variations: Top with grated orange rind mixed with coconut. Top with diced mint. Top with dollop of plain yogurt. Top with dollop of dairy sour cream.

Sesame Seed Snack

⅓ cup pure honey
½ cup pure peanut butter
1 Tbsp. peanut oil
3 Tbsp. powdered nonfat milk
2 Tbsp. soy flour or powder
1 Tbsp. lecithin granules
1 tsp. vanilla
½ cup chopped pecans
½ cup sesame seeds

Beat honey, peanut butter, and oil together with a wooden spoon. Gradually add dry milk, soy powder, and lecithin. Blend in vanilla, nuts, and seeds. Spoon batter into an oiled 10″ × 6″ pyrex pan. Pat mixture firmly and evenly. Bake for 20 minutes in 300° oven. Watch carefully as seeds can brown quickly. Makes 15 squares.

Sugarless Pumpkin Custard

1 Tbsp. flour or arrowroot powder
½ tsp. salt
1 Tbsp. ground coriander
2 Tbsp. ground pumpkin seeds
2 Tbsp. butter
2 cups pumpkin
3 Tbsp. molasses
3 eggs, beaten
1 can evaporated milk (13 oz.) or 1¾ cup whole milk
7 tablets artificial sweetener or other forms equal to 7 tsp. sugar
2 tsp. vanilla

Mix dry ingredients together in large mixing bowl. Stir in butter, pumpkin, and molasses. Combine beaten eggs, milk, sweetener, and vanilla and add to pumpkin mixture. Pour into buttered custard cups or pastry shell. Bake at 350° until firm or until knife inserted comes out clean.

Aunt Beulah's Custard

12 eggs, beaten
8 cups milk (2 quarts)
   (Canned evaporated
   milk may be used)

1 cup honey*
2 tsp. vanilla
¾ tsp. salt
nutmeg

Beat eggs slightly in large mixing bowl. Scald milk and pour into eggs. Stir in honey, vanilla, and salt. Strain custard into a 13″ × 9″ glass pan or individual custard cups. Place in a larger pan of hot water. Sprinkle nutmeg over the top. Bake for 35 minutes in 325° oven. When table knife inserted comes out clean, custard is done. Remove from hot water, cool, and then chill immediately.

*Diabetics may use an artificial sweetener suited to their taste.

Note for Senior Citizens:

This nourishing snack can be kept handy in the refrigerator, if covered, for one week. It's high in protein and calcium. Eat it with fruit or nuts to keep up your energy.

Hidden Sugars in Common Foods

FOOD	SERVING	AMOUNT OF SUGAR
Beverages		
Cider	6 oz.	4½ tsp.
Cola Drinks	6 oz.	4⅓ tsp.
Orangeade	8 oz.	5 tsp.
Root Beer	10 oz.	4½ tsp.
Seven-Up	6 oz.	3¾ tsp.

FOOD	SERVING	AMOUNT OF SUGAR

Cakes and Cookies

FOOD	SERVING	AMOUNT OF SUGAR
Angel or sponge cake	1 average piece	6 tsp.
Chocolate cake, two-layer, iced	1 average piece	15 tsp.
Coffee cake	1 average piece	4½ tsp.
Cupcake, iced	1	6 tsp.
Fruitcake	1 average piece	5 tsp.
Jelly roll	1 average piece	2½ tsp.
Pound cake	1 average piece	5 tsp.
Strawberry shortcake	1 average piece	4 tsp.
Brownie, no icing	1 average piece	3 tsp.
Fig newton	1 average piece	5 tsp.
Gingersnap	1 large	3 tsp.
Macaroons	1	6 tsp.
Oatmeal cookie	1	2 tsp.
Chocolate cookie	1	1½ tsp.
Chocolate eclair	1	7 tsp.
Cream puff, custard-filled, iced	1	5 tsp.
Donut, plain	1	4 tsp.
Donut, glazed	1	6 tsp.

Candies

FOOD	SERVING	AMOUNT OF SUGAR
Average chocolate bar (such as Hershey)	5 oz.	6 tsp.
Fudge	1 oz. square	4½ tsp.
Hard candy	1 piece	⅓ tsp.
Life Savers	1	⅓ tsp.
Peanut brittle	1 oz.	3½ tsp.
Gumdrop	1	2 tsp.
Marshmallow	1	1½ tsp.

FOOD	SERVING	AMOUNT OF SUGAR
Jam & Jellies		
Apple butter	1 Tbsp.	1 tsp.
Jam	1 Tbsp.	4 tsp.
Jelly	1 Tbsp.	4-6 tsp.
Orange marmalade	1 Tbsp.	4-6 tsp.
Pear butter	1 Tbsp.	1 tsp.
Maple syrup	1 Tbsp.	2½ tsp.
Dried Fruits		
Apricots, dried	4-6 halves	4 tsp.
Currants, dried	1 Tbsp.	4 tsp.
Dates, dried	3-4	4½ tsp.
Figs, dried	1½-2 small	4 tsp.
Prunes, dried	3-4 medium	4 tsp.
Raisins	¼ cup	4 tsp.
Canned Fruits		
Apricots	4 halves + 1 Tbsp. syrup	3½ tsp.
Applesauce, unsweetened	½ cup scant	2 tsp.
Fruit cocktail	½ cup scant	5 tsp.
Peaches	2 halves + 1 Tbsp. syrup	3½ tsp.
Prunes, stewed, unsweetened	4-5 med. + 2 tsp. juice	8 tsp.
Rhubarb, stewed	½ cup sweetened	8 tsp.
Stewed fruits, unsweetened	½ cup	2 tsp.
Fruit syrup	2 Tbsp.	2½ tsp.
Fruit Salad	½ cup	3½ tsp.

FOOD	SERVING	AMOUNT OF SUGAR

Canned Juices

Fruit juices, sweetened	½ cup	2 tsp.
Grapefruit juice	½ cup	3⅔ tsp.
Orange juice	½ cup	2 tsp.
Pineapple juice	½ cup	2 3/5 tsp.

Dairy Dishes

Chocolate, all milk	5 oz.	6 tsp.
Cocoa, all milk	5 oz.	4 tsp.
Eggnog, all milk	8 oz.	4½ tsp.
Ice cream cone or bar	1	5-6 tsp.
Ice cream soda	1	5 tsp.
Ice cream sundae	1	7 tsp.
Malted milk shake	1 10-oz. glass	5 tsp.

Miscellaneous Desserts

Custard	½ cup	4 tsp.
Apple pie	1 slice	12 tsp.
Berry pie	1 slice	10 tsp.
Butterscotch pie	1 slice	4 tsp.
Cherry pie	1 slice	14 tsp.
Custard pie	1 slice	10 tsp.
Coconut pie	1 slice	10 tsp.
Lemon pie	1 slice	7 tsp.
Mincemeat pie	1 slice	4 tsp.
Peach pie	1 slice	7 tsp.
Prune pie	1 slice	6 tsp.
Pumpkin pie	1 slice	10 tsp.
Raisin pie	1 slice	13 tsp.
Apple cobbler	½ cup	3 tsp.

FOOD	SERVING	AMOUNT OF SUGAR

Miscellaneous Desserts (continued)

FOOD	SERVING	AMOUNT OF SUGAR
Blueberry cobbler	½ cup	3 tsp.
French pastry	1 slice	5 tsp.
Jello	½ cup	4½ tsp.
Bread pudding	½ cup	1½ tsp.
Chocolate pudding	½ cup	4 tsp.
Cornstarch pudding	½ cup	2½ tsp.
Date pudding	½ cup	7 tsp.
Rice pudding	½ cup	5 tsp.
Tapioca pudding	½ cup	3 tsp.
Sherbet	½ cup	9 tsp.

CHAPTER FOUR

Nutrition Begins at Conception

God thought about me, and so I grew.—George Macdonald

At conception, that awesome moment when a squiggly, imperceptible male cell joins the larger egg cell of the female, a person enters the human family and nutrition begins.

This chapter is dedicated to all future mothers, because it is never too early for a woman to begin preparing her body to bear a child. During the period immediately following conception, when things can go "right" or "wrong," attention to proper nutrition can influence the child's entire life span.

A series of advertisements sponsored by the American Medical Association trumpets the slogan: "The time to start feeding your baby right is several years before it's born." By the time you've started to knit things, it could already be too late, the AMA ads emphasize.

"To nurture the baby growing inside her, a mother needs the strength that comes from years of good eating habits," says the ad. "During pregnancy, nutrition can have a direct, permanent effect on early brain growth. A seriously malnourished mother means a seriously deprived fetus. And that means a child born with less than full potential, physically and mentally."

If society can be educated and motivated to better dietary habits, says the AMA, then we can break a link in the vicious circle of poverty and ignorance that leads to malnutrition, to underdeveloped children, and full circle back to poverty and ignorance again.

The budding, fast-developing embryo cannot grow from nothing. Hour by hour, day by day it must receive nourishment from the mother who passes on to her baby what is received from the food she eats. A healthy mother provides all that the embryo needs; an unhealthy mother robs the new human being of the best cell development and causes all kinds of difficulties—major and minor—to arise. During pregnancy the problem of deformities, miscarriages, and retarded mental development are threats. Even if the baby hurdles these obstacles, more obscure troubles can develop later in life as the result of insufficient embryonic nutrition.

The cells tell

Each cell of the body has a unique makeup and distinct nutritional needs. Yet all of the cells must obtain their nourishment from the fluids that bathe them. We do not know precisely what each cell type needs or what happens when the needs are only partially met.

Perfect nutrition for cells throughout the entire body (each cell receiving exactly what it needs for maximum efficiency) is as rare as perfect health or perfect human conduct. It is human to err. But we should still try to make as few errors as possible. An expectant mother needs to be nourished with extraordinary care if the cells of her body (which in turn make up the cells of the embryo growing within her) are to be nourished at the highest level of efficiency. Extra care at this stage of development will return immense dividends later on—especially in terms of the brain, the most important organ of the body.

Give baby the best

The brain of a three-month-old baby weighs a little less than one pound—approximately one-tenth the weight of the tiny body. New brain cells continue to form until a child is one or two years old. However, the brain keeps increasing in size until the youngster is about eight years old. This growth is caused by enlarging brain cells and related structures of the brain. The brain of an adult weighs about three pounds.

Physicians are agreed that if the fetus is inadequately nourished the baby will be born with a smaller brain and have fewer brain cells than a healthy baby. Such a child will have learning problems and eventually, vocational problems. As adults, such children may be incapable of contributing to their society.

At the twenty-sixth annual Postgraduate Assembly of St. John's Hospital in Santa Monica, California, Myron Winick, M.D., told his colleagues, "Early malnutrition does lead to intellectual as well as other growth deficiencies in children, but there's still no simple answer as to how permanent these deficiencies may be."

Dr. Winick, a pediatrician who directs the Institute of Human Nutrition at Columbia University in New York City, added that even though a baby may be born deficient in nutrition, "we can reverse the negative effects of malnutrition by feeding [such] children adequately; but whether we can make up the whole deficit we don't know yet."

He said a child who is isolated from a stimulating intellectual environment will suffer the same kind of impairment that poor nutrition can bring. But the two—malnutrition and isolation—work hand in hand to rob a child of his full potential. "A poorly nourished child is often listless and not interested in his surroundings, no matter how enriched they have been made, so he loses ground mentally," Dr. Winick said.

Proper nutrition from conception through the first eighteen months of life is the ideal. These are the critical days during which the weight of the brain, the head circumference, the protein content, and the number and size of the brain cells are determined, Dr. Winick summarized.

In the fetal stage, the brain cells are dividing at the fastest rate. That's why it is important for an expectant mother to eat like a queen. Medical studies reveal that inadequate nutrition of the fetus produces a baby (if he makes it through birth alive) less capable of catching up in growth than a child malnourished only between the ages of twelve and eighteen months, for example.

Mrs. Gena Larson, in her book *Better Food for Better Babies and Their Families,* suggests a kind of "inner body cleansing." Numerous physicians prescribe a three-day juice diet or an exclusive diet of good natural food—without chemical preservatives—to purge out accumulated toxins and give the digestive organs a rest.

Author Larson suggests: "Three days of carrot and celery or zucchini juice, or of eating all the apples you wish, or the grape diet, both fruit and juice; or juicy, ripe watermelons if they are in season."[1]

Mrs. Larson also suggests mothers-to-be drink a concentrated acidophilus culture obtainable from a health food store for at least a three-month period after the initial cleansing to reestablish the friendly bacteria in the mouth, throat, and intestinal tract. Acidophilus is a natural culture of three specially developed strains of lactic acid bacteria: *lactobacillus Acidophilus, lactobacillus Bulgaricus,* and *lactobacillus Caucasicus.* These have been cultured in a manner that combines pure skim milk with a special type of yeast.

Milk is the natural food of lactic acid bacteria, since it supplies the lactose essential to optimum nutrition together with the vitamins and minerals that these bacteria require for good health. In addition, one-fourth cup of the liquid acidophilus mixed with 2 ounces apple or pineapple juice and taken shortly before mealtime, at least twice a day, will restore that wonderful feeling of radiant health. Or stir the acidophilus into buttermilk or yogurt and drink. Many dairies are now adding it to commercial milk.

A pregnant woman should also eat a balanced, varied diet adequate in calories as well as protein. A diet too low in protein will deplete protein in the mother's tissues. Research also shows that such a condition partially shuts down the transport of nutrients through the placenta. A calorie deficiency shuts down the transport mechanism, too.

Is the trouble and expense worth it for the heir? A medieval queen with limitless riches would have done it. You can, with a fraction of the expense or trouble.

Expectant mothers should refrain from taking any kind of over-the-counter drugs, even aspirin. Research has found this common remedy to be harmful to the fetus. There are many unknowns about other often-used drugs and their effects on the body and the embryo. Play it safe and decide you will not ingest anything that might be harmful to the marvelous new life within you.

Americans pride themselves on being the best-fed nation on earth, but there is a vast amount of improvement needed in the nutritional care of our young. The United States ranks fourteenth in cases of infant mortality and eighteenth in life expectancy for male babies.

A child who is not quite perfect is born in America every 73 seconds—1,177 more each day, nearly half a million a year. More than nine million youthful Americans under twenty-one are sufficiently impaired to require serious therapy.

Breast-feeding is best feeding

When it comes to comparing mother's milk with cows' milk for the newborn baby, nutritionists agree: mother's milk is far better for baby.

If for some reason it is impossible or unwise to breast-feed a baby, the doctor will advise the mother. Then perhaps together they can decide what is best for her baby. Mother's milk and cows' milk both have the same number of calories per ounce, but mother's milk contains less protein and more carbohydrates in the form of lactose or milk sugar.

Human milk is higher in polyunsaturates than cows' milk, but the fat content of both is about equal. Mother's milk is also lower in minerals—especially sodium and potassium, as well as calcium and phosphorus. However, the 2-to-1 ratio of calcium and phosphorus is ideal for the maximum calcium absorption that is so essential to a baby's developing bones and teeth.

Mother's milk has approximately twice the amount of vitamin A and niacin, but less thiamine and riboflavin. Mother's milk also has almost twice as much vitamin C and iron as cows' milk, but it still does not meet the recommended allowance for either. Most babies are born with enough iron stored in their livers to meet their needs until they begin eating other foods.

That much-needed iron came from the mother's own supply—another reason for her to make certain she is taking iron supplements while her baby is growing inside.

Recent studies indicate that many young American women are either quite low in iron or actually anemic. That's why most doctors prescribe iron supplements for expectant mothers.

Another interesting phase of our comparison here is that cows' milk—and most canned formulas as well—have three or four times as much salt as human milk. A normal baby can handle these amounts, but pediatricians ask, "Is it wise to include it?"

When large amounts of sodium are given to baby rats in early life they are more likely to develop hypertension (high blood pressure) in middle age. Pediatricians don't know if this applies to human babies or not, and they won't run the risk of experimenting on a new human being. But the addition of salt seems to be an unnecessary risk.

Our pediatrician enthusiastically encourages breast-feeding. He does not recommend it in cases of tuberculosis and similar diseases or if psychological apprehension makes it difficult for the new mother. "Unfortunately, our culture has made breasts a sex symbol instead of what God intended them to be," he said.

The La Leche League in Franklin Park, Illinois, states in its booklet *The Womanly Art of Breastfeeding:*

> The deepest, truest spirit of mothering grows as you experience the quick, strong feeling of affection so natural between a nursing mother and her baby; as you develop a sure understanding of your baby's needs, and joy and confidence in your own ability to satisfy them; and as you see the happy dividends from this good relationship as the baby grows. It is a spirit first sensed, gradually understood, finally realized fully by the mother who nurses her baby.

If it is impossible for you to breast-feed, it does not mean that you are not capable of warm mothering. To mother is more than to feed a child. Baby must be cuddled, rocked, talked to, listened to, gently soothed when necessary. In general, let the infant know he is loved, wanted, and enjoyed. Mothering is meeting a child's physical, mental, and emotional needs as he develops. If these aren't met with love and understanding he may have problems later.

When bottle-feeding, be sure to hold the baby—never prop up the bottle. If father is available allow him to have this sweet experience of cuddling and feeding the baby. Most men find this enjoyable and it helps them to get acquainted with their offspring. This can be immensely helpful if mother must tend another child at feeding time.

A twelve-member committee of specialists met in Washington, D.C., recently and drew up a list of recommendations concerning the benefits of breast-feeding, as follows:

1. The federal government, specifically the Department of Health, Education and Welfare, should initiate a campaign to inform parents of the advantages and techniques of breast-feeding. (The report called human milk "the ideal food for most infants.")

2. Infant formula cans and literature should not be permitted to carry such statements as "nearly identical to mother's milk." There are, in fact, significant differences, and such advertising and labeling is deceptive, the committee found.

3. Clinics and feeding programs under the Department of Agriculture should promote breast-feeding through promotional materials and through special supplemental food for lactating mothers.

4. Employers should adjust their policies to make it easier for working women to breast-feed their infants.

5. Hospitals, medical and nursing schools should evaluate their teaching of lactation and endorse breast-feeding whenever possible.

6. The National Institute of Health should sponsor

further research comparing breast-feeding with artificial formulas, with particular emphasis on psychological, denial, and allergenic effects.

7. The promotion of infant formulas in developing nations should be regulated, both by the local governments and by public pressure on the manufacturers, and programs to encourage breast-feeding—possibly including a lactation bonus of cash or food—should be established.

An advantage of a can

One advantage of a commercial infant formula is that it can be modified to meet special dietary needs. Premature babies often need a higher concentration of calories to guarantee enough energy for growth. Commercial formulas can be enriched from the usual 67 calories to as many as 100 calories per 100 milliliters to meet this need. A formula may come in handy for a "relief bottle" when the nursing mother must be away.

Breast-fed babies may add weight more slowly during the first six months of life, but at six months they grow more rapidly to catch up. Babies who are gaining too fast, or who have developed allergies, or who have certain other needs may require commercial formulas. But usually a baby will thrive on the milk provided by its mother and the experience is to be treasured by both parents.

Both of our boys were breast-fed. The experience strengthens the bonds of love between parents and children and, on the practical side, there's no work, no bottle to sterilize or milk to heat, and no possibility of error in mixing the formula!

> Suck, baby, suck! Mother's love grows by giving;
> Drain the sweet founts that only thrive by wasting!
> —Charles Lamb (1829)

And they thrive in another way: research finds that cancer of the breasts occurs less frequently in mothers who nurse.

Pre-highchair nutrition

Breast milk alone feeds the baby superbly for the first four to six months of life. After that, the baby's natural stores of nutrients will have run out. "Milk teeth" start to appear, signaling that the infant is ready for something more substantial than liquids. The muscles of baby's mouth are developed and his swallowing apparatus can handle semisolids.

Delaying semisolids beyond six months is shortsighted. By this time baby needs other foods to provide extra calories and protein, but most importantly vitamins and iron. Some pediatricians add cereal to the diet between four and six weeks. This is usually rice, oats, or barley— never wheat at this young age. Then when baby is eight weeks old, pureed fruit such as applesauce, bananas, pears, or peaches may be introduced. At twelve weeks mild-flavored pureed vegetables are recommended. The four-month-old can eat pureed meat and thrive on it. All the while these foods are being offered the baby's diet still is mostly milk, whether from the breast or bottle. Your doctor will advise you what is best for your baby's individual needs. Babies have different rates of growth and development, so their dietary needs may differ.

Between five and seven months a baby can be on three meals a day. Our sons were on the above program and were happy, healthy, and contented babies. They progressed to finger foods (from the four food groups) at nine months of age and were drinking easily from a cup at twelve months. This early exposure to varied foods has made them adventuresome eaters in their teen years.

If your little one is under the care of a medical doctor, the physician will chart a food program for you. He will probably prescribe vitamin-mineral supplements. We recommend medical supervision so that your baby will have the benefit of a supervised immunization program. This will prevent the potential danger of diseases and their complications. Children need not suffer from such miseries as measles and mumps in this modern day.

Prepare your own baby food

If any question lingers in your mind about whether to prepare your own baby food, the following information may help you come to the right decision.

Early in 1975 a government-sponsored committee of nutritionists, physicians, and citizen activists conducted a study on infant feeding practices. As a result a seventeen-page "White Paper on Infant Feeding Practices," sponsored by the Center for Science in the Public Interest, charged that manufacturers were adding such substances as sugar, salt, monosodium glutamate, spices, sodium nitrite (an element linked to cancer in animals) and large amounts of water to enhance flavor and appearance and thereby increase sales.

Exposure to sugar at such an early age, the study said, could lead to a preference for "junk food" during teen-age and adult years and a diet which might contribute to obesity-related diseases. This report led fifty-eight members of Congress, the Center of Science, and others to petition the Food and Drug Administration to require percentage ingredient labeling for all baby food products.

Instead of being honest, open, and cooperative, the spokesmen for the baby-food manufacturers refused to heed the warnings. Patricia Hausman, a research associate for the Center for Science in the Public Interest, found cooperation impossible. "Despite our repeated requests," she said, "Gerber, Heinz and Beech-Nut have refused to disclose how much sugar and starch are added to each of their products. Parents certainly have a right to know the composition of the foods they feed their children."

Dr. Ira Shannon, professor of biochemistry at the University of Texas, conducted laboratory analyses and discovered that Gerber's vanilla custard pudding derives 44 percent of its calories from added sugar, and Gerber's plums with tapioca derives 27 percent.

A representative of Gerber Products Co. strongly denounced the white paper. He said his company was unalterably opposed to the idea of ingredient labeling by proportion. "The formulation of products in a highly competitive business is privileged information and I think this is as true in the food industry as in any other industry," he declared.

He continued: "It's never been proved that bad eating habits come from infant feeding practices. Sugar is not an addictive product, and it does have some food value. And, for whatever it's worth, I believe there should be some pleasure in eating—why shouldn't a child have that opportunity, too? Haven't you ever had something you just plain enjoyed, regardless of whether or not it was good for you?"

Ms. Hausman found that sally easy to answer: "It has not been disproved that eating habits are formed in infancy—and until we do know for sure, we should be conservative and have the most nutritious foods possible. Infancy is one time when you can determine what an individual eats. Why not take advantage of this to insure good nutrition at an early age?"

Those statements by the Gerber spokesman alone are enough evidence for parents to shun commercial baby foods. He obviously doesn't know, or doesn't care about, the latest research on sugar and related diseases. We will repeat again: There is no nutritional value in sugar. It supplies energy but is incapable of nourishment. There is no reason to add refined sugar to the diet. We receive an abundance through our fruits, vegetables, and dairy products.

A representative of the Beech-Nut company said they would fight the proposal too. "Our mixture of raw ingredients is a secret formula that keeps our food from tasting the same as Gerber's or Heinz's," said the manager of consumer services. "I don't think any of the companies would go along with it."

You, the parent, have a right to know the proportion of nutrients in the baby food you buy. The baby food manufacturers appear to be more interested in their financial reports than in the health of our nation's infants. They are on record as not caring about consumers' wishes. You can register your outrage. Don't buy! Cook and make your own. Your baby will be safer and healthier for it.

In August, 1975, the Consumers Union produced an alarming report. In thirty-nine commercial baby foods they found insect parts, rodent hairs, and paint chips. These three contaminants were found in 25 percent of the foods tested, compared with about 10 percent of the samples tested in 1972. The filth was found in foods made by Gerber, Heinz, and Beech-Nut. Beech-Nut beef with vegetables and cereal was the worst offender. About twenty chips per jar were found.

They also discovered too much salt and sugar in the samples. It has been found that a high salt intake might predispose infants to hypertension as adults and that sugar could lead to tooth decay even in babies.

You don't have to pay for filth and such dietary danger. Buy a blender or a baby-food grinder, if you don't already have one. Invest a few extra minutes each day to give your baby pure food that you have prepared from your clean kitchen. You are not only giving the best for your baby but you are preparing him or her for a healthier life as an adult.

> Thank you for making me so wonderfully complex! ... Your workmanship is marvelous.... You were there while I was being formed in utter seclusion! You saw me before I was born and scheduled each day of my life before I began to breathe. Every day was recorded in your Book!
>
> —Psalm 139: 14, 15
> *The Living Bible*

THINGS TO DO

1. Start now to prepare for baby by eating wisely even before conception.

2. Since diet cannot always provide the maximum nutrients needed, take food supplements. Choose a competent physician for prenatal care, one who will prescribe vitamin-mineral supplements.

3. Give breast-feeding an enthusiastic and fair try.

4. Be at peace by filling your mind and heart with God's Word.

5. Prepare your baby's meals with fresh foods which the family eats, according to the recipes that follow. Processed baby foods can be harmful because of the glut of additives, sugar, and salt, and of questionable sanitary conditions in the manufacturing.

Fresh Apple Sauce

5 lbs. cooking apples (Jonathan, McIntosh, Rome Beauty, or Delicious)	1 Tbsp. lemon juice 3 Tbsp. honey

Wash, halve, and quarter apples. Do not peel. By leaving the skin on the apple you are retaining vitamins and minerals. Remove stems but leave seeds with the apples. Place apples in a 6 qt. pan or Dutch oven without water. Cover with tight lid. There will be beads of water on the apples from washing. Since apples have water of their own they'll produce their own juice. Start heat on medium high and as soon as vapor has been raised reduce heat to low. Don't be tempted to peek—you'll lose too much steam. Allow to cook at the low temperature for approximately 30-35 minutes. Apples will be tender to prick of fork. You will notice that 1-2 cups of juice were released from the apples. Remove and cool for about 5 minutes. Place apples a few at a time in a ricer and mash. You'll need to remove the skins and seeds as you mash through the apples. When all are mashed add the lemon juice and honey.

If you use Delicious apples you won't need any sweetener. Add the juice to the sauce. You'll have beautiful pink sauce with a marvelous flavor. If you have never eaten fresh apple sauce like this you're in for a taste thrill. You'll never buy it at the supermarket again. Baby and the rest of the family will be healthier for eating sauce prepared in this manner. If baby is tiny put applesauce through a sieve before serving.

Raw Applesauce

½ cup orange juice or   5 apples, peeled and sliced
   frozen juice concentrate
   for more vitamin C

Pour orange juice into blender and add apple slices slowly. Stop and start when necessary to stir. Serve immediately or chill. When baby is older, do not peel the apples.

Variations: Add plain yogurt and honey. Add cottage cheese. Add whipped cream for dessert. Garnish with a dollop of sour cream. Serve in paper cups for children's snack.

   For adults add:
     1 Tbsp. lemon juice
     1 tsp. lemon rind
     dash of nutmeg

Baby's First Foods

Cereal

Oatmeal
Cook old-fashioned rolled oats and puree in a baby-food grinder or in a blender with a little milk. Oats could be ground in the blender before cooking.

Fruit

Applesauce
Avocado
Banana
Peaches
Pears

These fruits should be ripe and pureed. If you must use canned peaches or pears, rinse off all the syrup before using. Baby should not have sugar.

Vegetables

Asparagus
Beets
Carrots
Corn
Green beans
Squash
Sweet potatoes
Cook vegetables for the family according to waterless method on page 244. Do not season during cooking. Remove baby's portion for one meal and puree in baby-food grinder or blender. (Then season vegetable with butter and salt for the rest of the family.)

Meat

Lamb
Veal
Chicken
Use meat served to family but choose the most tender meat for baby first. Do not season, but add a little meat juice or vegetable broth to make it moist and then puree. A little fruit may be added to make it easier to swallow.

Eggs

Begin with egg yolk only and not until baby is 6 or 7 months old. Hard boil and mix with cereal (be careful not to cook too long so yolk is dry). The egg white can be given later when there is less chance of an allergic reaction.

Cottage cheese

Puree with fruit of your choice.

Baby's Fruit Treat

1 avocado
1 pear
1 banana

¼ cup fruit juice or milk to allow blender to do its work.

Combine all ingredients and liquefy.

Vegetable-Yogurt Drink

½ cup yogurt
½ cup raw peas
½ cup cooked grated
  carrot

(The carrot is one vegetable that is more wholesome when cooked, as the carotene is released and assimilated.)

Place the ingredients in the blender and liquefy. Strain for small baby.

Limas and Corn

1 cup fresh green lima
  beans or frozen
  beans, cooked

½ cup cooked fresh corn, removed from cob or if frozen corn, cooked for 3 minutes.

Place beans and corn in blender. Add cream or milk to blend well. Strain for small baby.

Prune Whip

3 Tbsp. orange juice
1 cup yogurt
1 cup pitted prunes,

steamed tender
1 Tbsp. honey

Measure juice and yogurt into blender. Add several prunes at a time, mixing until all are blended. Mix in honey and serve immediately or chill. For small babies, mash mixture through a sieve to remove skins that might cause choking. Use raw prunes for older children.

SALAD IDEAS FOR TODDLERS

1. *Cooked* carrot grated (with nutmeg grater) and mixed with a little cream or milk. Add a tiny bit of fresh minced parsley.

2. Grated apple and grated *cooked* carrot mixed with a little yogurt and a tablespoon of orange juice.

3. Minced alfalfa sprouts with grated apple and tablespoon of orange juice.

4. Grated apple with cottage cheese and minced orange (remove membrane from oranges before cutting and mincing.)

5. Plain yogurt, mashed avocado, and grated apple.

6. Fresh minced tomatoes in cottage cheese.

CHILDREN'S SNACK SUGGESTIONS

Peanut butter, powdered milk, and honey mixed together make a yummy spread for bread, apples, and bananas and a stuffing for celery.

Cottage cheese stuffed in celery and sprinkled with crushed peanuts.

Carrot strips, green pepper strips, celery strips, and radishes dipped in plain yogurt that has been slightly seasoned with onion salt and minced parsley.

Cheese wedges with apple slices.

Fresh fruits of the season.

Banana chunks rolled in sour cream, then in crushed peanuts or coconut and served on toothpicks.

Cherry tomatoes and cheese chunks on toothpicks.

Raw asparagus spears dipped in a mixture of ½ cup mayonnaise, ¼ cup catsup.

Slice of cheese wrapped around a pickle and secured with a toothpick.

Little Red Apples: 3 oz. cream cheese softened to room temperature. Cut cheese into 12 cubes and roll into balls in buttered hands. Roll balls in minced chipped beef until well coated. Make an indention in the top, stick in a twig of parsley and insert a toothpick.

Homemade plain yogurt served with fruits in season and sweetened with a little honey.

Yogurt popsicles made with 1 cup yogurt and ½ cup fruit of your choice.

Frozen mixed vegetables in a dixie cup for munching.

Egg custard.

Pureed chicken livers, seasoned with onion salt, mayonnaise, and powdered mustard. Stuff into fresh, crisp celery. You may also add a little diced tomato.

Prunes, dates, dried apples, dried figs, etc.

See Snack Mix on page 62.

Homemade Peanut Butter

7-8 Tbsp. peanut oil or
  corn oil
3 cups fresh peanuts,
  shelled and skinned

salt to taste
6 Tbsp. powdered milk

Pour oil into blender and add peanuts and salt. Whiz at high speed, using rubber spatula to blend. Add powdered milk to butter to thicken a little and to make the protein from the peanuts a more complete protein.

Cashew Nut Butter

3 Tbsp. corn oil or   1½ cups cashews
   safflower oil   salt to taste

Pour oil into blender and add cashews and salt. Whiz at high speed using rubber spatula to blend. You can make it crunchy or smooth. This is delicious stuffed in celery or spread on apple slices for a snack. It is also high in unsaturated fat.

Raw nut butters may be made from almonds, Brazil nuts, cashews, filberts, pecans, peanuts, or English and black walnuts. Food grinders are available which will produce butter without the use of oil. Peanuts are an exception, but the Salton company makes a machine just for peanut butter. It's a good investment.

SCHOOL SANDWICH SUGGESTIONS

Chopped or ground chicken mixed with mayonnaise, pickle, and celery.

Mix ground ham with mayonnaise and crushed pineapple. Spread on rye, whole-wheat, or pumpernickel bread.

Whip peanut butter with powdered milk, orange juice, and chopped dates. Spread on oatmeal or whole-wheat bread.

Four hard cooked eggs, grated, ½ cup finely grated carrot, ¼ cup sugarless mayonnaise, ¼ tsp. salt, 1 sweet pickle finely diced. Spread on whole-wheat or oatmeal bread.

Tuna, sweet pickles diced, mayonnaise and a tsp. of onion. Spread on whole-wheat bread.

Turkey sliced thin or chopped with mayonnaise and spread on rye bread. Add alfalfa sprouts.

Two cups shredded natural cheddar cheese, ½ cup mayonnaise, 2 tsp. chives, and ¼ cup diced celery. Spread on whole-wheat bread.

Peanut butter, powdered milk, crushed pineapple, and grated carrots spread on whole-wheat bread.

Deviled ham mixed with thawed frozen peas and a little mayonnaise.

Chicken livers pureed and mixed with celery, mayonnaise, and minced onion.

Children should eat one third of their daily protein requirement at each meal. One third at breakfast, one third at lunch, and one third at supper. For children to do their best in school they must be fortified with an adequate breakfast.

Avoid processed lunch meats because of dangerous chemicals.

CHAPTER FIVE

How Firm Is Your Foundation?

Dust thou art...—Genesis 3:19

The windows of the South Bend-to-Chicago jet dripped with moisture as we circled O'Hare for forty-five minutes awaiting clearance to land. The mood of the passengers matched the gray skies outside. Suddenly a teen-age girl in a soiled jeans pantsuit stood up and began wandering back the aisle toward us, searching from side to side for an empty seat. We had inadvertently been seated in the smoking section in a row with the only available seat, so she paused and asked, "May I sit here?"

"Of course," we replied.

"I need a cigarette and I can't smoke up there," she explained.

In the conversation that followed during our holding pattern aloft, we learned that the eighteen-year-old girl had been released from jail the previous day and was heading home to Minneapolis. To our questions about prison food she replied that the juveniles in her ward breakfasted on strong coffee, donuts, and other baked goods. They lunched on canned peaches, spaghetti, white bread, and coffee. Supper included a sandwich, salt, two cookies, and more coffee.

She seemed surprised when we urged her to select more nutritious foods now that she was out of prison. Her eating habits had been little better before she ran away from home. Could poor diet be one reason she couldn't get along with her mother? Could lack of a good nutritional foundation be part of the cause of her trembling hands, her fear of meeting her loved ones at the other end of the line, her pallor and pimples and rebellious attitude?

Psychiatrists, endocrinologists, and nutritionists have discovered that there is a relationship between our mental stability and emotional health and the food we eat. That food—bone of our bone and flesh of our flesh—is the subject of this detailed chapter.

Each person enters the world with distinctly different nutritional needs. No creature is "normal"; each has a unique anatomy. The vital bodily organs are different in size, shape, and performance. Athough many of our characteristics are genetically determined, body chemistry may differ widely among individuals in the same family. There are so many variables within the complicated processes of the body that no set of nutritional rules will fit all people. So we must learn more of the "biochemical individuality" that characterizes each person.

The brilliant biochemist Dr. Roger J. Williams, in his book *Biochemical Individuality,* published by the University of Texas, offers hope in his statement: "Nutrition applied with due concern for individual genetic variations, which may be large, offers the solution to many baffling health problems."

Following is an abbreviated listing of bodily elements and their functions in keeping you healthy. They include:

Proteins, Vitamins, Macrominerals, Microminerals, Carbohydrates, Fats, Enzymes, and Water.

We have set forth the recommended daily allowances (RDA) (see end of chapter) only as a guide. Your individual requirements may be greater. Learn to know and understand your body. After eating certain foods, do you feel great or do you feel nauseated? Does coffee make you jittery? Do you have a sinus headache an hour after eating chocolate? You may have blamed the headache on another cause.

Observe how your body reacts to food; make sure you're eating a wide variety. Never be satisfied with poor performance of your marvelous machine. Study the charts and plan your program.

Proteins

You are a splendid tower of more than 100,000 different kinds of protein. Everything that shows—hair, nails, skin, eyes—is essentially protein. The muscles you use to move your eyes across these lines are protein tissues. Internally, too, you are essentially protein. Your body is put together with some thirty trillion cells, each special type requiring its own individual kind of protein.

While plants are the original protein source, a proper combination of animal and vegetable foods is required to produce proteins of a higher nutritional value than plants alone are able to supply. The protein from plants and animals must be changed into different forms before it can be used in human cell tissues. This is the special trick of those master magicians, the enzymes. They free amino acids for use by the body, so that it can promote digestive chemical reactions that split large food proteins and reassemble their amino acids into usable human building blocks.

Complementary Proteins

It is important that we learn to combine certain foods that complement each other to increase the protein value. This will eliminate the need for so much meat in the diet. Many of our traditional food combinations are good examples. Our Spanish menus include corn tortillas plus rice and beans—an excellent combination.

Perhaps we serve pea soup with grilled cheese sandwiches. We use milk on our granola. Legumes should be eaten with grains because they have amino acids that grains do not have. Together you have more usable protein. Any of these foods are less usable to our body if eaten alone, but when eaten together supply the amino acid combination that provides a complete protein. All the amino acids must be present simultaneously in order for the body to benefit.

Here are combinations that you should plan to serve together, using the strongest food groups:
1. Milk + grains (corn + soy; rice; wheat; wheat + peanuts)
   Milk + nuts and seeds
   Milk + beans
   Milk + potatoes
2. Nuts and seeds + legumes
                  + dairy products
                  + grains
3. Grains and legumes
   Rice + legumes
   Corn + legumes
   Wheat + legumes

Vitamins

More people than ever are supplementing their diets with vitamins. Overworked soil, insecticides, radical food processing procedures, and seasonal variations all combine to interfere with the original nutrients the natural food had to offer.

The United States government allows 2,800 different chemical substances to be used to increase our food's shelf life. There are approximately 8,000 additional chemicals in our natural environment. Some are poisonous, others are not. All are unnatural to the human body.

Organic foods, grown on properly nourished soil and not exposed to chemical fertilizers, pesticides, sprays, or other pollutants, have become popular. Today they are easily found and are eaten by purists willing to pay for the extra cost.

Why is there resistance to vitamin supplements?

When you ask your physician whether you should supplement your diet with vitamins, he will probably answer in one of three ways: (1) They surely won't hurt you, (2) They aren't really necessary, or (3) I can give you medication which will make you feel better more quickly.

Remember, most drugs suppress the symptoms of your malady while vitamins and minerals help to remove them. The route of balanced nutrition is longer, but it leads to more satisfactory results.

Vitamins manufactured in the United States are labeled according to the U.S. RDA (Recommended Daily Allowances). These have the force of law behind them. They are legal definitions kept firmly under the thumb of the Food and Drug Administration (FDA).

Vitamin A

The oldest vitamin on record is vitamin A—the substance that helps to develop and sustain hair, eyes, glands, teeth, skin and gums.

Infection can destroy it in the blood; increased dosage is needed when infections or injury plague the body. Long periods of infection produce deficiencies. So does a lot of mineral oil if taken regularly to overcome constipation. This habit prevents the absorption of all fat-soluble vitamins, including A, D, and K.

Never diagnose your own vitamin A deficiencies. Dosage that is too large may be harmful since the body stores A like D. The U.S. RDA is 5,000 International Units (IU). (See chart at the end of this chapter for sources.)

The Vitamins B

A lack of vitamins in the B family (commonly called the nerve vitamins) can result in skin and hair disorders, changes in the mouth, eye, and reproductive glands, or abnormalities in the utilization of other nutrients. Stress can cause a greater need for water-soluble B vitamins.

The eight B vitamins as we know them are:

Vitamin B_1 or thiamine: Stressful situations (including surgery), exposure to cold, and the experiences of adolescence, pregnancy, or aging can increase the need for B_1. Excessive cooking reduces the amount of B_1, as does an abundance of carbohydrates. The U.S. RDA of B_1 is 1.5 mg.

Vitamin B_2 or riboflavin: A deficiency of this vitamin can lead to pellagra or other diseases such as glossitis (inflammation of the tongue), anemia, and cheilosis (lesions in the corner of the mouth). Again, psychological stress and infection are enemies of riboflavin. U.S. RDA is 1.7 mg.

Niacin or nicotinic acid (B_3): Deficiencies in niacin cause trouble with the skin, bowels, and nervous system. Severe weight-reducing strategies and alcohol are the worst offenders in robbing the body of niacin. Results: headaches, stomach pain, irritability, and insomnia. Mental distraction and a red, furry tongue are also symptoms. U.S. RDA: 20 mg.

Vitamin B6 (pyridoxine): Metabolism errors in babies can be corrected with heavy doses of vitamin B6. B6 is needed for the oxidation process required in the metabolization of alcohol, and alcohol use can deplete it. B6 helps stop vomiting during pregnancy. Women taking oral contraceptives require more B6 (as well as C, B12, and folic acid). People taking antidepressant drugs and victims of some types of anemia are helped by B6. The U.S. RDA is 2 mg., and there is little chance that you can take in too much.

Pantothenic Acid: Together with vitamin A, pantothenic acid is involved in the work of the adrenal glands and helps prevent damage that stress can cause the body. It releases energy from food, and vitally affects behavior and brain functions. Sufferers from inadequate pantothenic acid may experience fatigue, apathy, headaches, nausea, insomnia, and abdominal discomfort. U.S. RDA is 10 mg.

Biotin: Biotin deficiencies can result in drowsiness, aches in muscles, and numbness to certain areas of the body. Also eczema-like rashes can develop, along with pallid skin and disturbances of the stomach and intestines. The intestines of both man and animals produce biotin. U.S. RDA is 0.3 mg.

Folic Acid: This substance is also called "folacin." Pregnant women and those on oral contraceptives should take folacin as a supplement. Alcoholics with anemia also must be treated with folacin. Folic acid helps to overcome fatigue, appetite loss, shortness of breath, and swelling of mouth membranes. It also keeps the immunological defenses of the body strong. U.S. RDA is 0.4 mg.

Vitamin B12: Associated with vitamin B_{12} are the labels *cyanocobalamin* and *hydroxocobalamin.* Without B_{12} the body is open to pernicious anemia, which also can result in the degeneration of nerves, fostering neuritis, poor eyesight, and the inflammation of the gastrointestinal tract. It may even result in mental confusion leading to psychosis. Vitamin B_{12} is active in the production of the nucleic acids DNA and RNA, and is also involved in the strategic functions of important enzymes.

Never take any of the B vitamins alone. Any supplement should be balanced with the other B vitamins so that they can work together.

Vitamin C

The body needs vitamin C to heal its wounds, integrate its capillaries, and develop blood vessels, bones, and other tissues. Vitamin C is active in the development of cell glue—the sticky substance inside a cell that holds it together. Vitamin C is irreplaceable in the metabolism of certain areas since many transactions inside the cell cannot proceed without it.

Vitamin C is resident in the endocrine glands and influences the function of the adrenal cortex. It helps to banish fatigue, lethargy, sluggish appetite, and aching joints. It even works as a kind of cosmetic to improve skin texture. This water-soluble vitamin should be a major part of any supplement, taken preferably in time-released capsules.

Probably more has been written about vitamin C than about any other single nutrient for the body. Each fan of the vitamin has his own tales of its wonders. Since your body may not assimilate vitamin C as quickly as another person's, and since toxic amounts (overdoses) are practically unknown, vitamin C added to your supplemental diet is excellent. The only side effect we've been able to discern from large doses is a touch of diarrhea.

An unnatural frequency of colds or sore throats may indicate a deficiency in vitamin C. Cigarette smokers burn up 25 milligrams of the vitamin with every cigarette and need supplements beyond the RDA. Stressful conditions on the job or in the home make your need for vitamin C greater; so does a respiratory weakness.

Dr. Linus Pauling, two-time winner of the Nobel Prize, noted that from 1,000 to 2,000 milligrams a day are needed to resist infectious diseases such as the common cold. People with colds should take from 500 to 1,000 milligrams each hour until the symptoms disappear. Use caution in cases of kidney ailments.

Oranges are a traditional source of vitamin C, eaten whole or taken as juice.

> Whole orange: (with fiber content) ....75 mg. C
> Frozen: 1 cup reconstituted juice ....112 mg. C
> Fresh: 1 cup squeezed from orange .....129 mg. C

The ideal way to obtain vitamin C is to eat the entire orange. Underneath the peel is a layer of white pulp called albedo, a soft substance that is very high in bioflavonoids. It also offers fiber, which is necessary for good health.

Vitamin D

Growing children need more of this "bone and teeth" vitamin than older people, but it can be toxic in both age levels if taken in excess. The body manufactures its own vitamin D through sunlight when seasons allow it. Vitamin

D permits the absorption of calcium and phosphorus to take place in the intestines. Obtain it naturally in live fish oils. Years ago parents made their children swallow cod liver oil as a standard dietary supplement. Today the bone vitamin is part of multivitamin preparations. Milk and babies' formulas are fortified with 400 International Units per quart. Deficiency is rare. The U.S. RDA is 400 IU.

Vitamin E

Vitamin E functions mainly as an antioxidant, protecting other materials against oxidation or helping to stop physiological changes produced by oxidation. It serves as an antioxidant in holding back the oxidation of unsaturated fatty acids in the body's tissues.

Foods with good supplies of vitamin E include wheat germ, fresh beef liver, fruits and green leafy vegetables, mayonnaise, nuts, vegetable oils, and corn, peanut, and soya oils. The U.S. RDA is 30 IU and there is no danger of overdose.

Vitamin K

Often called the "blood vitamin," K is the coagulation substance. Its very name comes from *Koagulations-vitamin.* It permits the blood to clot by helping the liver to synthesize prothrombin. A balanced diet usually contains adequate supplies of the blood vitamin. Normal intestines supply the added amounts. Nature stores it in alfalfa sprouts and green, leafy vegetables. It is found also in pork liver, cows' milk, and vegetable oils. The vitamin is a fat-soluble ingredient, although water-soluble brands have been manufactured. They are useful in injections during bleeding problems.

Minerals

Our second listing among food elements includes the nuts-and-bolts of the body—minerals. You can't live without minerals, although vitamins usually take center stage. Minerals that the body requires in large doses are called "macrominerals." Those found in smaller doses (just a trace) are called "micronutrients" or "trace minerals."

Macrominerals

The macrominerals include:

Calcium: Your body has more calcium than any other single mineral—two or three pounds in teeth and bones. It is found in milk products, green leafy vegetables (except spinach and chard), citrus fruits, and dried peas and beans.

Phosphorus: Your body's tissues require it and a good diet will supply all you need. It is found in meat, poultry, fish, eggs, and whole-grain foods. Vegetables and fruit have it in short supply.

Sodium and chloride: These elements combined make ordinary sodium chloride (table salt), however each has a special function to perform in the body.

Potassium: This mineral resides in the fluid inside the cells of your body. Along with sodium, it helps to regulate the volume of fluids. Prolonged diarrhea robs the body of potassium. So do diuretics causing excessive urination. Potassium is present abundantly in bananas, oranges, and other foods. Orange juice has been recommended by the American Heart Association for use in low-salt diets, providing much potassium and almost no sodium.

Sulphur: Another mineral present in all body tissues is sulphur. It is a part of two vitamins—thiamine and biotin. Life is not possible without it.

Microminerals

Although present in reduced quantities, the "trace" minerals: cadmium, cobalt, copper, fluorine, iodine, iron, manganese, magnesium, molybdenum, nickel, selenium, tin, vanadium, and zinc, are also essential for good health. With certain exceptions, the human body cannot store micronutrients. Unfortunately, it has more of a tendency to store bad minerals like lead than the good ones which need constantly to be replenished.

Poor eating habits and stress are the twin culprits in robbing the body of its essential minerals. But remember: too much of a good thing can lead to trouble. Trace elements are essential only in small quantities and can be poisonous in overloads. A laboratory analysis of a clipping of hair from the scalp can determine what mineral or minerals you may lack.

Carbohydrates

Carbohydrates (starches and sugars) provide the chief source of energy for most people. Cereals (wheat, rice, corn, oats), sorghum, and tuber roots (potatoes, beets, yams, and turnips) are loaded with starches. Carbohydrates can be found in beans, peas, and other legumes as well as in sugars such as table sugar (sucrose), fruit sugar (fructose), and milk sugar (lactose).

The main source of carbohydrates is plants. However, animals provide small amounts through lactose (milk). All meat, except for liver, has no carbohydrates.

Sugars are found in honey, syrup, and table sugar. The average American eats a total of 126 pounds of sugar annually: 105 pounds of cane and beet sugar and 21 pounds of corn syrup.

The brain needs glucose, another sugar, to operate, but

the brain manufactures all it needs from starch and proteins. The sugar on the table—beet or cane—is virtually pure sucrose. It contains only empty calories. It's the same with brown sugar and raw sugar. They have the same effect on diabetics; however, people with this disease can tolerate natural sugars in most foods as long as their intake is limited to a diabetic's proportion.

Americans tend to eat too many carbohydrates. The consequence is obesity, increasing heart disease, and low blood sugar, which is becoming a national scourge.

Your body gets sufficient amounts of carbohydrates in a balanced diet. You would be better off eating no sugar at all.

Fats

Fifth in our list of food components is the grouping loosely called "fats." Any study of fats must include oils and cholesterol as well. The modern diet of Americans is fattier than ever, but not necessarily more healthful. Affluence introduces a wide variety of heavy food, and sometimes it is our undoing.

Fat to the biochemist is a *lipid.* It offers such basic health benefits as energy, heat conservation, vitamin transport, hunger gratification, lubrication, the manufacture of body cells, shock absorption, nerve calming, aid to vital functions, and a supply of essential fatty acids, along with pleasurable taste. Fats are necessary for good health, but polyunsaturated fats instead of saturated fats are recommended to help prevent heart attacks and strokes.

The specter of cholesterol

The word cholesterol comes from the Greek word *chole* for "bile" and *sterol* for "solid." It is found in headlines of newspapers, in research reports, and on the lips of millions of Americans facing the grim killer heart disease.

As a substance it is a tasteless, odorless, white fatty alcohol found in all animal fats and oils. The body produces its own in the liver, with some assistance from other organs. It's not all bad. The body needs cholesterol for the synthesis of bile acids required for digestion and absorption of fats in the intestine, and the manufacture of steroid hormones and vitamin D.

So, be wise. Avoid the dangers to your heart through correct use of fats, oils, and cholesterol.

Enzymes

The essential biological catalysts that make life possible are those curious agitators called enzymes. They are added to a hundred commercial products—from bread dough to meat tenderizers—and effect chemical changes in the body without which we could not live.

Enzymes are a special type of catalyst because they are biological in origin. They are made from protein, and the biochemical processes they trigger are vital to every living cell. Enzymes are found in all living organisms. They are the activators, overseers, and regulators of molecules: the universal agents of life.

Water

Although this nutrient isn't listed among our five components, water is such a vital element that it must not be overlooked. From earliest history, supplies of water have been guarded and preserved as carefully as foodstuffs. It's possible to live for weeks without food, but lack of water kills much more quickly. The longest recorded survival of life on the ocean without drinking water is eleven days.

About seven-tenths of the body is water. Blood is 90 percent water. Even muscles contain from 80 to 90 percent water. This fluid is so essential to life that a loss of less than 20 percent leads to a painful death.

To keep the body's water supply at a normal level, the average person takes in about a ton of water each year—either as the water he drinks or in the food he consumes. Water carries the food and takes the wastes away from the living cells of even the most complicated living animals and plants. Drink plenty.

How firm is your foundation? Knowing what your body needs each day is the first step in supplying these vital nutrients. Hang loose, eat wisely, stay slim, get exercise, stop smoking, and accentuate the positive.

THINGS TO DO

1. Learn to understand and know your own individual needs. If you are under unusual stress your requirements are greater for the B vitamins and vitamin C.

2. Buy only the freshest fruits, vegetables, seafood, poultry, and meat. Eat the *whole* fruit for maximum vitamin, mineral, and fiber content. Eat the vegetables raw when possible. Include in your diet more poultry and fish and moderate amounts of lean beef.

3. Eat a protein-rich breakfast. We should consume one third of our daily protein requirement at breakfast. This is necessary to keep children alert in school and adults thinking efficiently.

4. Eat a wide variety of foods. Never overcook your food. Many B vitamins and vitamin C are lost if foods are cooked

too long. Deep-fat frying should be a rarity. Avoid deep fried food in restaurants. When fat is not changed often a chemical reaction in the fat can cause it to become carcinogenic.

5. Even the best choices often fall short of maximum nutrition requirements. If you are not energetic, considering your age, you probably need vitamin-mineral supplements.

Make your night out nutritious

We all object to spoiled meat, burned toast, and a chef's hair in our soup. But how many customers in restaurants ever give a thought to more harmful excesses like rancid fat, lettuce sprayed with preservatives, and croutons made from leftover table rolls?

Ironically, tests have shown that often the quick/cheap burger chains offer cleaner food than some high-priced "quality" restaurants. So when you eat out, try to know your restaurant.

Here are a few simple rules that will help you get the most nourishment for your nickel, or stay on a prescribed diet.

1. Order meats that are individually cut, uncamouflaged by breading and rich sauces.

2. Avoid deep-fried fish, meat, and potatoes. The hot fat is often too old and therefore rancid. You cannot detect when oil is rancid. Also, fat reheated at high temperatures is changed chemically and can bring about a carcinogenic reaction in your body.

3. Soups often contain leftover meat and vegetable tidbits which have lost most of their nutritional value. They are often oversalted and enhanced by monosodium glutamate and other flavor stimulators. Recent research indicates that monosodium glutamate causes headaches in certain individuals.

4. Fresh green, fruit, or fish salads are usually a good menu choice.

5. When possible, order fresh vegetables such as sliced tomatoes. Some restaurants will allow substitutes like fresh tomatoes or cottage cheese in place of french fries, for example.

6. Get additional protein by ordering milk (low-fat or buttermilk preferably) instead of coffee, tea, or colas.

7. Always inquire about alternative choices. Remember, your waiter or waitress should desire to please you, the valuable customer.

8. Because excessive water, heat, and oxidation destroy vitamins and minerals, cafeteria-style steam tables offer particular hazards for vegetables. In such situations, choose fresh vegetable salads to get the most nutrition.

9. Train your taste buds to enjoy fruit for dessert—fresh when possible—instead of rich pies and cakes. Good dessert selections are baked custard, baked apples, or cheese and nuts.

10. Take good care of your waiter and your waiter will take good care of you.

The Richest Sources of Vitamin A Are:

Food	Approx. Amount	International Units
Lamb	2 slices	74,000
Beef liver	3½ oz.	53,400
Chicken liver	3 pieces	32,200
Carrots	1 cup cooked	18,130
Carrots	1 cup raw	13,000
Spinach	1 cup	11,800
Collards	1 cup	11,700
Mustard greens	1 cup	10,500

Food	Approx. Amount	International Units
Sweet potatoes	1 medium	8,900
Kale	1 cup	8,000
Cantaloupe	½ medium	6,000
Broccoli	1 cup	5,100
Beet greens	1 cup	5,100
Butter/fortified margarine	½ cup	3,700
Tomatoes, raw	1 medium	2,600
Milk, whole powdered	1 cup	1,160
Eggs	2	1,180

The United States Recommended Daily Allowance 5,000

The Richest Sources of Vitamin B_1 Are:

Food	Approx. Amount	Milligrams
Powdered brewer's yeast	¼ cup	5.2
Sunflower seeds	½ cup	1.8
Wheat germ	1 cup	1.4
Rice polish	½ cup	.9
Soy flour	1 cup	.9
Pork roast	3 oz.	.8
Brazil nuts	½ cup	.6
Brown rice	1 cup	.6
Whole wheat	1 cup	.6
Soybeans	1 cup	.4
Yellow cornmeal	1 cup	.4
Beef liver	3½ oz.	.3
Dry lima beans, cooked	1 cup	.3
Peas, fresh	1 cup	.3

United States Recommended Daily Allowance (RDA 1.5)

The Richest Sources of Vitamin B_2 Are:

Food	Approx. Amount	Milligrams
Torula yeast	¼ cup	6.0
Lamb	2 slices	5.1
Kidney, braised	3½ oz.	4.8
Pork	2 slices	4.4
Calf liver	1 slice 3½ oz.	4.2
Chicken livers	3 medium	2.4
Powdered whole milk	1 cup	1.5
Wheat germ cereal	1 cup	.9
Wheat germ	1 cup	.5
Cottage cheese	1 cup	.6
Almonds	½ cup	.6
Turnip greens	1 cup	.6
Eggs	2	.3
Broccoli	1 cup	.2
Collards	1 cup	.2
Kale	1 cup	.2
Parsnip	1 cup	.2
Spinach	1 cup	.2

United States Recommended Daily Allowance (RDA 1.7)

The Richest Sources of Vitamin B_3 (Niacin) Are:

Food	Approx. Amount	Milligrams
Torula yeast	¼ cup	40
Lamb liver	2 slices, 3½ oz.	24.9
Pork liver	2 slices, 3½ oz.	22.3
Beef or calf liver	1 lg. slice, 3½ oz.	16.5
Rice polish	½ cup	14
Sunflower seeds	½ cup	13.6

Food	Approx. Amount	Milligrams
Powdered brewers yeast	¼ cup	12.9
Chicken livers, fried	3 med.	11.8
Tuna, canned	3 oz.	10.9
Kidney, braised	3½ oz.	10.7
Swordfish, broiled	1 steak	10.3
Halibut, broiled	3½ oz.	9.2
Rice, brown	1 cup	9.2
Peanuts, roasted	⅓ cup	8.6
Turkey, roasted	3½ oz.	8.0
Peanut butter, natural	⅓ cup	7.9
Duck, domestic	3½ oz.	7.9
Chicken, roasted	3½ oz.	7.4
Mackerel, canned	3 oz.	7.4
Chicken, broiled	3 oz.	7.0

United States Recommended Daily Allowance (RDA   20)

Sources of Vitamin B6 (pyridoxine):

Beef liver, kidney, pork loin and ham, leg of veal, fresh fish, cabbage, bananas, avocados, walnuts, prunes, raisins, wheat germ, soybean flour, brown rice, and split peas. B6 is present in only moderate amounts in milk and eggs.

Sources of Pantothenic Acid:

Lamb, kidney, broccoli, beef, kale, avocados, split peas, lentils, lima beans, walnuts, cashews, egg yolk, wheat bran, and oats. Milk has only sparce amounts.

Sources of Biotin:

Egg yolk, many fresh vegetables, liver, and kidney.

Sources of Folic Acid (folacin):

Kidney, liver, round steak, wheat germ and other wheat products, yeast, green, leafy vegetables, Swiss chard, asparagus, black-eyed peas, lima and red kidney beans, and orange juice.

The Richest Sources of Vitamin C Are:

Food	Approx. Amount	Milligrams
Guava	½ cup	1,000
Orange juice, fresh	8 oz.	129
Green sweet pepper	1 large	120
Papaya, fresh	½ med.	112
Broccoli, steamed	1 cup	105
Strawberries, frozen	1 cup	93
Turnip greens, steamed	1 cup	90
Grapefruit juice	1 cup	84
Watercress leaves & stems	1 cup	80
Collards, steamed	1 cup	75
Orange, whole	1 med.	75
Grapefruit, fresh 5″ dia.	½ cup	72
Desiccated liver, defatted	¼ cup	70
Cantaloupe	½ med.	65
Brussel sprouts, steamed	1 cup	60
Kale, steamed	1 cup	60
Mustard greens, steamed	1 cup	60
Cabbage, steamed	1 cup	53
Cabbage, as coleslaw	1 cup	50

United States Recommended Daily Allowance (RDA   45)

Pregnant   60 mg.

Lactating   80 mg.

FOOD AND NUTRITION BOARD, NATIONAL COUNCIL RECOMMENDED DAILY

Designed for the maintenance of good nutrition

	Age (years)	Weight (kg)	Weight (lbs)	Height (cm)	Height (in)	Energy (kcal)[b]	Protein (g)	Fat-Soluble Vitamins			
								Vitamin A Activity (RF)[c]	Vitamin A Activity (IU)	Vitamin D (IU)	Vitamin E Activity (IU)
Infants	0.0—0.5	6	14	60		24 kg × 117	kg × 2.2	420[d]	1,400	400	4
	0.5—1.0	9	20	71		28 kg × 108	kg × 2.0	400	2,000	400	5
Children	1-3	13	28	86	34	1,300	23	400	2,000	400	7
	4-6	20	44	110	44	1,800	30	500	2,500	400	9
	7-10	30	66	135	54	2,400	36	700	3,300	400	10
Males	11-14	44	97	158	63	2,800	44	1,000	5,000	400	12
	15-18	61	134	172	69	3,000	54	1,000	5,000	400	15
	19-22	67	147	172	69	3,000	54	1,000	5,000	400	15
	23-50	70	154	172	69	2,700	56	1,000	5,000		15
	51+	70	154	172	69	2,400	56	1,000	5,000		15
Females	11-14	44	97	155	62	2,400	44	800	4,000	400	12
	15-18	54	119	162	65	2,100	48	800	4,000	400	12
	19-22	58	128	162	65	2,100	46	800	4,000	400	12
	23-50	58	128	162	65	2,000	46	800	4,000		12
	51+	58	128	162	65	1,800	46	800	4,000		12
Pregnant						+ 300	+30	1,000	5,000	400	15
Lactating						+500	+20	1,200	6,000	400	15

[a]The allowances are intended to provide for individual variations among most normal persons as they live in the United States under usual environmental stresses. Diets should be based on a variety of common foods in order to provide other nutrients for which human requirements have been less well defined.

[b]Kilojoules (k J) = 4.2 × kcal.

[c]Retinol equivalents.

[d]Assumed to be all as retinol in milk during the first six months of life. All subsequent intakes are assumed to be half as retinol and half as ß-carotene when calculated from international units. As retinol equivalents, three fourths are as retinol and one fourth as ß-carotene.

ACADEMY OF SCIENCES—NATIONAL RESEARCH DIETARY ALLOWANCES,[a] Revised 1974
of practically all healthy people in the U.S.A.

	Water-Soluble Vitamins						Minerals					
Ascorbic Acid (mg)	Folacin[f] (mg)	Niacin[g] (mg)	Riboflavin (mg)	Thiamine (mg)	Vitamin B6 (mg)	Vitamin B12 (mg)	Calcium (mg)	Phosphorus (mg)	Iodine (mg)	Iron (mg)	Magnesium (mg)	Zinc (mg)
35	50	5	0.4	0.3	0.3	0.3	360	240	35	10	60	3
35	50	8	0.6	0.5	0.4	0.3	540	400	45	15	70	5
40	100	9	0.8	0.7	0.6	1.0	800	800	60	15	150	10
40	200	12	1.1	0.9	0.9	1.5	800	800	80	10	200	10
40	300	16	1.2	1.2	1.2	2.0	800	800	110	10	250	10
45	400	18	1.5	1.4	1.6	3.0	1,200	1,200	130	18	350	15
45	400	20	1.8	1.5	2.0	3.0	1,200	1,200	150	18	400	15
45	400	20	1.8	1.5	2.0	3.0	800	800	140	10	350	15
45	400	18	1.6	1.4	2.0	3.0	800	800	130	10	350	15
45	400	16	1.5	1.2	2.0	3.0	800	800	110	10	350	15
45	400	16	1.3	1.2	1.6	3.0	1,200	1,200	115	18	300	15
45	400	14	1.4	1.1	2.0	3.0	1,200	1,200	115	18	300	15
45	400	14	1.4	1.1	2.0	3.0	800	800	100	18	300	15
45	400	13	1.2	1.0	2.0	3.0	800	800	100	18	300	15
45	400	12	1.1	1.0	2.0	3.0	800	800	80	10	300	15
60	800	+2	+0.3	+0.3	2.5	4.0	1,200	1,200	125	18+[h]	450	20
80	600	+4	+0.5	+0.3	2.5	4.0	1,200	1,200	150	18	450	25

[e]Total vitamin E activity, estimated to be 80 percent as *a*-tocopherol and 20 percent other tocopherols.

[f]The folacin allowances refer to dietary sources as determined by *Lactobacillus casei* assay. Pure forms of folacin may be effective in doses less than one fourth of the recommended dietary allowance.

[g]Although allowances are expressed as niacin, it is recognized that on the average 1 mg. of niacin is derived from each 60 mg. of dietary tryptophan.

[h]This increased requirement cannot be met by ordinary diets; therefore, the use of supplemental iron is recommended.

Comparative Nutritive Values

BREAKFAST
Each 700 calories

Wholesome	*Inadequate*
half grapefruit	3 hotcakes with butter
2 eggs	and syrup
3 oz. ham	1 cup coffee with sugar
1 slice buttered toast,	and cream
whole grain	
1 glass milk	

Furnishes:		*Furnishes:*
45 gm	PROTEIN	.8 gm
40 gm	FAT	.30 gm
40 gm	CARBOHYDRATES	.100 gm
700	CALORIES	.700
460 mg	CALCIUM	.65 mg
760 mg	PHOSPHORUS	.100 mg
7 mg	IRON	.2 mg
17 ug	IODINE	.4 ug
4200 USP Units	VITAMIN A	1400 USP Units
0.8 mg	THIAMINE (B$_1$)	.0.4 mg
1.07 mg	RIBOFLAVIN (B$_2$)	.0.18 mg
15 mg	NICOTINIC ACID	.0.6 mg
50 mg	ASCORBIC ACID	

In comparison with the above 700-calorie inadequate breakfast, the 700-calorie wholesome breakfast furnishes more than ...

. Five times as much protein
. Seven times as much calcium
. Seven times as much phosphorus
. Three times as much iron
. Four times as much iodine

. Three times as much vitamin A
. Six times as much vitamin B_2 (riboflavin)
. Twice as much vitamin B_1 (thiamine)
. Twenty times as much nicotinic acid
. Fifty times as much ascorbic acid

Comparative Nutritive Values

LUNCH
Each 655 calories

Wholesome	*Inadequate*
Vegetable soup	Ham sandwich
Shrimp salad	Coke or other soft drink
1 slice whole-grain bread/butter	Slice of pie
1 glass buttermilk	
1 apple	

Furnishes:		*Furnishes:*
28 gm	PROTEIN	11 gm
27 gm	FAT	21 gm
75 gm	CARBOHYDRATES	105 gm
655	CALORIES	655
370 mg	CALCIUM	75 mg
440 mg	PHOSPHORUS	120 mg
4 mg	IRON	0.6 mg
34 ug	IODINE	1.4 ug
1930 USP Units	VITAMIN A	420 USP Units
0.26 mg	THIAMINE (B_1)	0.070 mg
0.53 mg	RIBOFLAVIN (B_2)	0.10 mg
3.0 mg	NICOTINIC ACID	2.5 mg
10 mg	ASCORBIC ACID	1.0 mg

In comparison with the above 655-calorie inadequate lunch, the 655-calorie wholesome lunch furnishes more than...

. Twice as much protein
. Four times as much calcium
. Three times as much phosphorus
. Six times as much iron
. Twenty times as much iodine
. Four times as much vitamin A
. Four times as much thiamine (B₁)
. Five times as much riboflavin (B₂)
. Ten times as much ascorbic acid

Comparative Nutritive Values

DINNER
Each 890 Calories

Wholesome	*Inadequate*
4 oz. tomato juice	Spaghetti and meatballs
Green salad with vinegar dressing	Green salad with French dressing
Roast beef, 6 oz.	French bread and butter
Baked potato w/1 sq. butter	French pastry
Half of cantaloupe	Coffee with sugar and cream
1 oz. cheddar cheese	
Glass buttermilk	

Furnishes:		*Furnishes:*
70 gm	PROTEIN	28 gm
30 gm	FAT	40 gm
85 gm	CARBOHYDRATES	105 gm
890	CALORIES	890
600 mg	CALCIUM	175 mg
860 mg	PHOSPHORUS	320 mg
10 mg	IRON	4 mg

45 mg	IODINE	11 mg
4900 USP Units	VITAMIN A	1900 USP Units
0.84 mg	THIAMINE (B$_1$)	0.26 mg
1.40 mg	RIBOFLAVIN (B$_2$)	0.29 mg
16 mg	NICOTINIC ACID	4.5 mg
90 mg	ASCORBIC ACID	10 mg

In comparison with the 890 calorie inadequate dinner, the 890-calorie wholesome dinner furnishes more than...
. Twice as much protein
. Five times as much calcium
. Twice as much phosphorus
. Twice as much iron
. Four times as much iodine
. Twice as much vitamin A
. Three times as much thiamine (B$_1$)
. Three times as much riboflavin (B$_2$)
. Four times as much nicotinic acid
. Nine times as much ascorbic acid

(1,000 milligrams $=$ 1 gram)
(10,000 micrograms $=$ 1 gram)
USP United States Pharmacopoeia

Used by Permission
International College of Applied Nutrition, La Habra, California.

Chicken Cacciatore
(Crock Pot Cooking)

1 3-lb. chicken, cut into pieces or 3 lbs. of your favorite cut
½ cup flour
¼ cup olive oil (no substitute here)
1 medium onion, chopped
1 large green pepper
1 clove garlic
2 cups fresh tomatoes or your own frozen or canned
1 bay leaf
6 sprigs parsley
1 sprig fresh thyme or ½ tsp. dried whole leaf thyme
2 tsp. salt
½ cup fresh sliced mushrooms
½ tsp. Kitchen Bouquet (optional) stirred in with mushrooms

Thoroughly rinse chicken and use paper towels to pat dry. If on low-fat diet remove skin from chicken. Dredge each piece of chicken in flour. Heat olive oil in skillet and quickly brown* chicken. While chicken is browning place onions, green pepper, garlic, tomatoes, and seasonings in pot. Transfer chicken to pot and pour any remaining oil onto chicken. Cover, set on low, and cook 5-7 hours. Meat should be tender. Stir sauce around chicken and add mushrooms. Cover again and cook until mushrooms are heated through. Serve with hot buttered spinach spaghetti.

*If you're in a hurry the browning step can be eliminated. Stir the olive oil into the tomatoes and proceed without using the flour.

Irish Lamb Stew
(Crock Pot Cooking)

1 clove garlic, grated
1 medium onion, chopped
3 Tbsp. corn oil
4 or 5 carrots, scrubbed, sliced about ¼″ thick
3 medium potatoes, peeled and cut into ¾″ thick bite-size pieces
3 Tbsp. fresh parsley or 2 tsp. dried

1½ lbs. lamb stew meat
¼ tsp. pepper
¼ tsp. ginger
½ tsp. oregano
1 tsp. salt
2 cups boiling water
2 tsp. instant bouillon
1 small pkg. frozen peas

In frying pan over medium heat sauté garlic and onion in oil. Place carrots, potatoes, and parsley in slow cooker. With slotted spoon transfer onions and garlic to pot.

Place carrots, potatoes, and parsley in slow cooker. With slotted spoon transfer onions and garlic to pot.

Brown lamb in hot pan with the leftover oil.

Sprinkle all the seasonings over the onions and then stir into vegetables with a wooden spoon. Add the browned meat. Pour one cup boiling water into empty frypan and stir, scraping all the browned drippings. Measure the other cup of water and stir in the bouillon. Add to skillet and blend. Pour liquid over lamb, cover cooker, set on low, and cook for 8-9 hours. Last half hour add peas.

Norm's Favorite Oysters
Pennsylvania Dutch Style

⅓ cup melted butter
4 cups crushed crackers or bread crumbs
1¼ tsp. salt

¼ tsp. pepper
1 pint oysters
2 cups oyster juice and milk

Melt butter and add to crumbs. Stir in salt and pepper. Add alternate layers of crumbs and oysters in a buttered casserole. Pour liquid over contents of dish and top with crumbs. Bake in 375° oven for 30 minutes. Serves 6.

Swiss Steak
(Crock Pot Cooking)

1 medium onion, peeled and sliced into thin rings
1½ to 2 lbs. round steak
½ cup flour
3 Tbsp. oil
1 cup water

2 cups nonfat milk
¼ tsp paprika
¼ tsp. pepper
½ tsp. salt
2 Tbsp. cooking sherry

Place onions on the bottom of slow cooker or crock pot Cut steak into individual pieces. Dredge in flour and brown in oil in hot skillet. Remove and place on top of onions. Add remaining flour to drippings in skillet and brown.

Add water, milk, seasonings, and sherry. Stir until thick and smooth. Pour over meat, cover cooker, set on low, and cook 8 to 12 hours. Serve with brown rice, peas, and carrots, green salad, and milk or tea.

Aunt Helen's Sweet and Smoky Chicken

1 frying chicken cut up, or your favorite pieces
1 tsp. hickory smoked salt
    OR
1-2 Tbsp. bar-B-Q liquid smoke

Sauce:
¼ cup minced onion
½ cup catsup, homemade
½ cup maple syrup
¼ cup cooking oil
2 Tbsp. prepared mustard

Rinse chicken and pat dry with paper towel. Sprinkle salt over chicken or use pastry brush to cover each piece well with liquid smoke. Place chicken in baking dish with skin side up and bake covered with foil for one hour in 350° oven. Remove from oven and take off foil. Cover each piece with the sauce and return to oven uncovered. Reduce heat to 300° and bake one more hour. Serves 4.

Baked Chicken Breasts

5 chicken breasts, cut in half to make 10 serving pieces
2 cups sour cream
2 tsp. salt
1 tsp. paprika
½ tsp. ground cayenne
1 tsp. sweet basil leaves
2 Tbsp. soy sauce
2 fresh garlic cloves, peeled and crushed through garlic press
2 cups crisp bread crumbs or dressing mix

With a sharp knife, completely bone the chicken. Also remove skin. With a paper towel blot both sides of chicken and remove any little bones that are clinging. Place chicken in a shallow glass baking dish 9″ × 13″. Mix sour cream and seasonings and pour over chicken. Gently turn each piece so it is well coated. Cover tightly with foil and chill overnight.

Place crumbs in plastic bag and crush thoroughly with a rolling pin. Transfer to a shallow dish. Remove chicken from the refrigerator and dip into the bread crumbs, shaping each piece with the fingers. Sprinkle any remaining crumbs on top. Return to pan and refrigerate at least 1½ hours longer. When ready to cook uncover and bake in moderately slow oven, 325° for 1 hour 15 minutes. Remove chicken to hot platter. Garnish with watercress or parsley.

Meal Suggestion:
Serve with brown rice, green salad, yellow vegetable, and fruit. Makes 10 servings.

Creole Proverb:
Ka poul bwe dlo, li pa blie Bo-Die.
"When a chicken drinks water it doesn't forget to raise its head in thanks to God."

Chicken-Fried Liver

1½ lbs. fresh beef liver
3 Tbsp. lemon juice
¼ cup flour
1 tsp. salt
¼ tsp. paprika
¼ tsp. pepper

¼ cup milk
1 egg, slightly beaten
1½ cups finely rolled
  bread crumbs or cracker
  crumbs
vegetable oil

Rinse liver under running water. Pat dry with paper towels and sprinkle with lemon juice. Combine flour and seasonings in pie pan and coat each piece of liver well. Combine milk and egg in flat dish; dip liver into mixture and then coat with crumbs. Heat oil in skillet and sauté liver for about 5 minutes on each side. Serve hot.

Vege-Taco

3 Tbsp. butter
1 bunch green onions,
  diced
4 small zucchini squash,
  thinly sliced (after
  brushing clean, taste to
  see if skin is mild—if
  bitter, peel off skin)
½ green bell pepper,
  minced

1 cup fresh mushrooms,
  diced
¼ cup cashews, crushed
1 ripe avocado, diced
2 cups natural cheddar
  cheese, grated
bowl of alfalfa sprouts
1 doz. tortillas

Melt butter and sauté vegetables together for 5-7 minutes. Stir in nuts. Place in bowl. Fry tortilla quickly in hot corn oil. Drain. Place helping of hot vegetables onto tortilla followed by cheese, avocado, and alfalfa sprouts. Fold over and enjoy.

Chile-Avocado Supreme

2 4-oz. cans Ortega chiles
½ lb. grated cheddar
  cheese
½ lb. grated Jack cheese
2 beaten egg yolks
¾ cup evaporated milk
2 Tbsp. flour

½ tsp. salt
¼ tsp. chili powder
2 egg whites
Sauce:
1 cup tomato sauce
2 ripe tomatoes
½ ripe avocado, peeled

Rinse chiles and cut open lengthwise to remove all seeds, as they are very hot. Drain on paper towels. Line a 10″ × 6″ pyrex pan with half of the chiles. Reserve others for next layer. Sprinkle cheddar cheese over chiles. Layer remaining chiles on cheese. Cover with layer of Jack cheese. Mix yolks, milk, flour, and seasonings together. Beat egg whites until stiff but not dry. Fold into milk mixture and pour over chiles and cheese. Bake for 45 minutes at 325°. Remove from oven. Heat sauce and then pour over top. Peel tomatoes, slice, and arrange over sauce. Add avocado slices and place under broiler until bubbly. Remove and let set for about 5 minutes. Cut into 8 pieces and serve immediately.

Meal suggestion:

Serve with hot brown rice, tossed green salad with sliced zucchini, radishes, and a grated carrot. Use dressing of choice.

Mex Spaghet

3 lb. beef chuck roast
2 Tbsp. corn oil
1 clove garlic
1 tsp. salt
½ tsp. black pepper
3 cups water
1 medium chopped onion
3 Tbsp. cornstarch
3 Tbsp. water
1 7-oz. can whole Ortega chiles, chopped
2 cups fresh or canned tomatoes, chopped
1 Tbsp. fresh or dried cilantro, chopped
1 tsp. chili powder
chopped meat
4 or 8 oz. spaghetti (wheat or spinach made by Buitoni is higher in protein)

Brown roast in hot oil in Dutch oven or other large pan with lid. Slice fresh garlic in strips and insert into meat with the help of a knife. Sprinkle meat with salt and pepper. Reduce heat to low. Add water and onion and cover. Simmer for 3 hours or until meat is tender. When done remove meat to a plastic chopping board and cut into bite-size pieces. Skim fat off broth in pan. (If time permits, the broth can be placed in freezer to allow fat to harden, and then skimmed off.) Mix cornstarch and water together until smooth and add to remaining liquid in pan. Stir and simmer until thickened. Add chiles, tomatoes, cilantro, chili powder, and chopped meat. Simmer 15 minutes while you cook the spaghetti according to package directions. Personal preference on the amount of spaghetti or number of people to be served can determine whether you cook 4 or 8 oz. Blend into beef mixture and serve. Serves 8-10.

Brown Rice Salad

1 cup brown rice
2⅔ cup water
1 tsp. salt
1 Tbsp. oil
1 cup diced celery
⅓ cup pecans, chopped or
  whole
1 cup fresh pineapple
  chunks

1 Tbsp. sliced green onion
2 cups diced cooked
  turkey, chicken or ham
½ cup mayonnaise
¼ cup sour cream
1 Tbsp. lemon juice
¼ tsp. salt
dash of sweetener

Bring salted water to a boil. Add rice and oil. Cover with a tight lid and cook over low heat until rice is tender and all the water is absorbed, approximately 50 minutes. Chill. Add celery, nuts, fruit, onion, and meat. Toss together.

Beat mayonnaise, sour cream, and seasonings together. Pour over rice mixture and blend well. Keep refrigerated until serving time. Serve on fresh greens* and garnish with tomato wedges or green grapes.

*Fresh greens can be lettuce, watercress, spinach leaves, or another favorite green. Use your imagination.

Rice Pudding
(Crock Pot Cooking)

2 cups cooked brown rice
2 cups milk
2 eggs, slightly beaten
¼ cup honey
1 Tbsp. melted butter

2 tsp. vanilla
¼ tsp. salt if rice has already
  been salted
¼ tsp. cinnamon
½ cup raisins

Mix all ingredients in a one-quart casserole. Pour ½ cup water in crock pot or slow cooker. Place uncovered dish onto a metal band from canning jar or a metal trivet placed in bottom of pot. Cover with pot lid and turn heat to high. Cook 2 hours. Serve warm or cold with whipped cream slightly sweetened with honey. Serves 4-6.

CHAPTER SIX

Tomorrow's Meat for a Burgeoning World

God never sendeth mouth but he sendeth meat.

—Heywood, *Proverbs*

Early in 1971 our lives took on a new dimension with the formal incorporation of Food for the Hungry by Dr. Larry Ward. Norman was invited to serve on the board; later Virginia became temporary office manager at Dr. Ward's request.

The facts we learned about world hunger were sobering, but the ambitions of the new organization were bright and optimistic.

At mealtime, we read to our two sons reports about hunger and thirst and famine in faraway places. It seemed that we could hear the hoofbeats of the black horse of famine as it thundered across our modern world with increasing speed.

We also read comments like those of comedian Lenny Bruce who charged: "I know in my heart by pure logic that any man who claims to be a leader of the church is a hustler

133

if he has two suits in a world in which most people have none."

It became easy to appropriate a portion of our income for food for the hungry...easy to let the wardrobe stand at one suit...easy to pray for the less fortunate. Imagine 12,000 people starving to death every day!

The global picture can be likened to ten children seated at a dinner table ready to divide up the food. Three of the youngsters, looking their healthiest, pile their plates high with substantial portions of most of the milk, eggs, meat, and fish. The children eat their fill and discard the rest. Two other children at the table finish their plates, getting enough—just enough—for basic nutritional requirements. The other five children are left without enough food. Three are lethargic, sickly, swallowing small portions of bread and rice. Two can't even do that. They eventually die from dysentery and pneumonia, too weak to care much.

Food for the Hungry's initial strategy was (1) to meet disaster emergencies quickly, without red tape, (2) to stockpile food in various parts of the world where it would be readily available in case of emergencies, and (3) to foster small farm units structured within the culture of the country.

It has become clear that a large portion of the sophisticated technology of the Western world won't work in countries socially and culturally out of step with such wasteful harvesting.

It is clear also that the grain-cattle-meat cycle robs the world of vegetable protein which, if not fed to cattle, could keep many people alive. Next time you select an eight-ounce steak at the supermarket's meat counter, look around. There are forty-five starving people standing with empty bowls which could have been filled with the grain it took to grow that piece of meat.

Protein derived from animal sources is too expensive for

most families in the global community of four billion people. Soon animal protein may be unavailable at any price. Production of meat protein requires a costly double cycle: the crops draw their nourishment from soil, the animals eat the crops and turn it into protein, the animals are then slaughtered and eaten to provide protein that originated with the crops for the diet of man.

The Chinese cow

Vegetable protein can be just as nutritious as animal protein. At the top of the list among vegetables offering body-building protein is the soybean. This complete food has played such a major role in the Chinese diet for centuries that it has been tagged "The Chinese cow."

There is no single perfect food containing all nutrients in sufficient quantities to supply all bodily needs alone. Milk is probably the nearest, but even this "perfect" food needs nutritional cohorts to keep the body properly fueled.

The soybean (when sprouted) is as nearly perfect as the milk of a cow, while also supplying iron and vitamin C. Soybean milk can be substituted for cows' milk when an individual is allergic to the dairy version.

So far, soybeans have been used mainly in the animal feed industry. We predict that the day will come when this amazing "meat" will be the mainstay of the human diet around the globe. More abundant use of soybeans in the human diet will bring the eater better health, longevity, and economy—three objectives of every conscientious homemaker.

George M. Strayer, formerly with the American Soybean Association, points to the period of World War II as a time when the United States doubled and redoubled its production of soybeans. It was the logical means of increasing edibles inexpensively at a critical time of shortages worldwide. Today, Mr. Strayer points out, the United States is the world's largest producer of soybeans.

The plant is native to China, its name first recorded in the Chinese *materia medica* "Pon Tsai Gong Mu," authored by Emperor Sheng-Nung, the "god farmer," in 2383 B.C.

North Americans must eat meat, milk, eggs, and cheese to get the type of protein the Chinese obtain by eating soybeans. It might be safely stated that the Chinese nation exists today because of the use of the soybean as a food.

The vegetable came to North America in 1804, but no large-scale production was begun until 1924. In 1971 soybean farmers produced more than one billion bushels harvested on 43 million acres. Thus the raising of soybeans is the fastest growing U.S. industry of the past decade. It is the number one cash crop in U.S. agriculture.

Since creation, man has had a continuing tension between population growth and his supplies of food. If the present population curve continues to spiral upward, the global census in 2000 A.D. will total 7.5 billion people. Author and researcher Philip Chen estimated in 1973 that there were four billion acres of cultivatable land on the globe. Divide this by four billion inhabitants and you can see how much land there is for each person.

Tomorrow we'll be hungry

An estimated 2.5 acres are said to be required to clothe and feed an individual adequately. Then what must the future hold with global population rising by two percent each year?

Even before World War II, two-thirds of the world's population were continually undernourished, according to John Boyd Orr, UN food expert. Today more than 12,000 people die every twenty-four hours from starvation. What is the prospect for tomorrow?

Obviously, new sources of protein must be found and tapped if the multiplied billions in tomorrow's world are to be fed adequately. It's unlikely that enough new acres can be successfully tilled to care for the increased human load on planet earth, due to problems with climate, topography, or soil. Large-scale irrigation schemes also can be fickle.

Every suggestion for increasing the world's food supply has limiting factors, including birth control, improved fertilizers, soil conservation, insecticides, cold- and drought-resistant strains of grains, concentrated food forms such as yeast and algae, etc.

One logical solution seems to be plowing up of pasture lands for grain crops and sowing soybeans rather than crops of lower food value.

Dr. T. L. Bywater of the University of Aberdeen early suggested the first solution in an article for *Science News Letter,* August 30, 1950. In it he declared: "To provide food for the world's population now having its greatest growth in history, the amount of land used for direct human food crops will probably be increased, while that for the support of livestock will be reduced."

Naturally, hilly land unsuitable for cultivation can be left in pasture for grazing animals as the most productive way to garner its protein. But as far back as 1944 a scientist of Chinese nationality stated:

"As long as animals are, like men, dependent on the green plant for food, animal products are always more expensive than plant products. In obtaining his food indirectly from the plant via the animal, man has to pay the price of the middleman. In order that every country may reach a dietary standard similar to that of the United States, the animal products of the world would in turn require a twofold increase in the area of pasture land as existent today. And this increase in pasture land would cause a diminishing of crop land corresponding to about fifteen times its size, since one acre of land devoted to the production of grains yields six to seven times as much food energy as that devoted to the raising of dairy cattle."[1]

Dr. Robert S. Harris of the Massachusetts Institute of Technology stated at the International Conference on Vitamins held in Havana before American-Cuban relations deteriorated: "Both the vegetarian type and the carnivorous type of diet can adequately feed mankind. It does not matter whether the calcium comes from milk or tortilla, whether the iron comes from meat or tampala, whether the niacin comes from liver or peanuts, whether the tryptophane comes from eggs or soybeans, or whether the calories come from wheat or rice, so long as these nutrients are available."

The tests tell

Is a vegetarian diet really adequate? A survey conducted by Dr. Mervyn G. Hardinge of the College of Medical Evangelists and Dr. Frederick J. Stare of Harvard University, published in the *Journal of Clinical Nutrition*, 2:73 (1954), indicates that vegetarians can be as healthy as anyone.

These medical researchers studied persons eating three types of menus: (1) lacto-ovovegetarian, a diet of plants plus eggs and milk but no meat, either fish or fowl; (2) vegetables alone, excluding milk and eggs; and (3) no vegetables at all, eating instead milk, eggs, meat, and foods originating from plants.

All three dietaries, Doctors Hardinge and Stare discovered, came within the limits of the daily allowances of nutrients recommended by the National Research Council. Height, weight, red cell count, hemoglobin concentration, and blood pressure were all pretty much the same among the 201 people participating in the survey.

Levels of cholesterol among the three types of adults varied widely, however. The last group, the non-vegetarians, had the highest blood cholesterol of all. The second group, pure vegetarians, had the lowest count. The first group fell in between.

The researchers summed up their report by stating:

"Despite the fact that the differences observed between the dietary choices of the two groups [vegetarian and non-vegetarian] were small, certain advantages of even the commonly practical lacto-ovovegetarian regime were evident:

"1. Constipation was less common in the vegetarian than in the nonvegetarian groups.

"2. Approximately half of the nonvegetarian expectant mothers had swelling of the ankles and were on salt-free or salt-restricted diets, while among the comparable lacto-ovovegetarian expectant mothers only one had slight ankle swelling and none were on salt-free or salt-restricted diet.

"3. Acne, though common in all adolescent groups, was more severe among the nonvegetarian youths.

"In addition to these points, the reader will recall those previously mentioned, namely the lower blood cholesterol levels found among the vegetarians than among non-vegetarians and the fact that the 'pure' vegetarians approached more closely to their ideal weight.

"The cumulative evidence of this study—restricted as it necessarily was—indicates not only an adequacy but a possible superiority of the average lacto-ovovegetarian diet over a nonvegetarian diet."[2]

Since a vegetarian diet suffices so adequately, the soybean stands tall among its green and leafy associates as a handy backstop in cases of weather failure that would damage livestock feed or bring shortages of other food.

The influence of diet in cases of coronary disease is quite significant. George Dock, Jr., writing years ago said in the

November 1946 issue of *The Reader's Digest:*

"Hospital death records indicate that among executives and professional men coronary disease causes nearly 25 percent of all death. The higher toll of coronary disease among men than among women was explained until recently by the tension and worry of business life. Now a different answer is suggested by microscopic studies of the coronary arteries of many persons of both sexes who died from various causes, at ages ranging from a few hours after birth to seventy years. If these findings are confirmed by wider research, the strain of making a living has much less to do with coronary death among men than the combination of two other factors—the structure of their arteries and the food they eat."[3]

Coronary disease and arteriosclerosis are caused in part by cholesterol taken from meat, eggs, and milk. But the soybean contains phytosterol instead of cholesterol. You can eat as much of this "meat" as you wish and not run the risk of coronary disease and arteriosclerosis.

The soybean is not only an inoffensive main dish but one that actually aids in the cure of disease. An enterprising physician once prescribed for his patients suffering from hypercholesterolemia (high cholesterol in the blood), not a low-fat diet but rather the opposite—one that was actually high in cholesterol—in addition to soybean phospholipids which the food industry markets as lecithin.

A total of 122 people volunteered for the high-fat regimen and ate raw liver and raw brains and other food rich in cholesterol. Ninety-nine of them ate a teaspoon of lecithin at every meal. The twenty-three others did not. When the tests were taken the 79 percent of the patients who took the lecithin enjoyed a dramatic decrease in blood cholesterol. The patients who did not take it had no lessening of blood cholesterol.

Conclusion: a diet of soybean lecithin can correct hypercholesterolemia. Soybean lecithin can also serve to reduce dangers from coronary disease and arteriosclerosis.

Other benefits

Because the soybean contains high protein levels and low starch content it is beneficial in the diets of diabetic patients. Somehow it reduces the percentage of sugar passed into the urine of diabetics who eat the foods usually prescribed for diabetes.

The soybean has the unique ability to create and sustain a favorable intestinal flora. Thus it rids the body of offensive germs which pollute our intestinal tracts and cause colitis and other acute maladies like skin rashes and headaches.

Soybeans are a blessing for people with food allergies. They have been known to clear up pimples, eczema, rashes, and other skin irritations. The soybean is a beneficial food for persons suffering from arthritis, rheumatism, and allergy-caused asthma. The soybean works well in these cases because it eliminates the need for meat, eggs, and milk, lessening the inflammatory activities of the skin.

You are using the soybean now in ways of which you might not be aware. Most soybean oil today goes into a variety of food products. Shortening takes the most soybean oil; margarine is next. Other food products such as salad oils, salad dressings, and cooking oils come in third. Soybean oil is used in bread, cakes, and cookies; prepared mixes such as cake, biscuit, pie dough, sweet dough, potato chips, nuts, and many other fried foods; canned fish and soups; candies of various kinds.

Whether you are healthy or ill, rich or poor, plain or gourmet, the soybean can become for you and for the world a source of nutritious and tasty food for all seasons.

THINGS TO DO

1. Educate yourself about the versatile soybean.

2. Include lecithin in your dietary program.

3. Use the soybean as a meat substitute. Save money by using this high quality protein vegetable.

4. Consider using soy milk in cases of suspected allergy to cows' milk.

5. Treat your family to new soybean dishes, including those on the following pages.

Dry Soybeans

Sort

Before cooking, remove any discolored, cracked, or shriveled beans. After sorting, measure beans and wash thoroughly. One cup dry soybeans will yield 2½ to 3 cups cooked beans.

Soak

Use 4 cups water for 1 cup of dry beans. To soak them quickly, boil beans 2 minutes, remove from heat and let stand 1 hour. Drain. Or, boil beans 2 minutes and let them stand overnight in the refrigerator to prevent fermentation. Drain.

The soybean has an anti-enzyme factor that can inhibit the assimilation of another protein. For this reason beans should be soaked overnight and *drained* so the water-soluble enzyme or inhibitor is removed. This is obviously contrary to what you do with other beans. With ordinary beans you soak overnight, but cook in the same water.

Boil

Add 1 tsp. salt for each cup of dry beans. Simmer beans covered with water in a covered pan. Add water if necessary during cooking. To reduce foaming, add 1 to 2 tsp. oil to the cooking water. Follow the prescribed cooking time.

Bake

Follow recipe.

Store

Cooked soybeans may be stored about 1 week. They also may be frozen.

Soy Flour

Soy flour from the bean comes in three types:

1. Full-fat flour, which contains more than 35 percent protein and about 20 percent fat—all of the fat present in whole beans. This is the type available in stores and used in this book.

2. Low-fat flour, which contains about 6 percent fat and nearly 45 percent protein.

3. Defatted flour, which has had the fat removed by hexane extraction. This flour contains less than 1 percent fat and about 50 percent protein.

Soy flour has a variety of uses and advantages in baking:
- It keeps baked products from becoming stale.
- It provides rich color and moistness.
- It increases nutritive value of food.

Use 1 or 2 Tbsp. of soy flour in the bottom of measuring cup before filling with all-purpose flour or other flours. Products containing soy flour brown more quickly, so baking time or temperature should be adjusted slightly.

Store soy flour in a cool, dry place. Because of its high fat content, it may become rancid if stored at too high a temperature.

Soy Milk

Soy milk is available commercially in dry, concentrated and ready-to-use forms. Instructions for preparing, serving, and storing are on the package. Soy milk may also be prepared at home.

Commercial soy milk is often fortified with vitamins and minerals to approximate the composition of cows' milk.

Soy milk may be used in place of cows' milk in most recipes. Due to the flavor difference between soy and cows' milk, you may prefer to use half soy milk and half cows' milk.

To prepare about 2 quarts of soy milk, use 1 pound (2½ cups) dry soybeans. Sort and wash beans thoroughly.

Using 2 quarts of water, soak beans overnight or use the 2-minute-boil method (p. 142). Drain soaked beans and discard the soaking water. Remove the skins from the beans if you wish to use the bean mash or pulp after the milk is made.

Using 3 quarts of water, grind the soaked beans in a blender. Place part of the beans and enough water to cover in blender container; grind until very fine (about 2 minutes). Repeat until all beans have been ground and the 3 quarts of water have been used.

Strain ground beans through two layers of cheesecloth into a large kettle. Wring as much liquid from the mash as possible. (To use mash, see below.)

Boil the soy milk for 30 minutes, stirring occasionally to prevent scorching. It is necessary to cook the milk thoroughly to destroy a substance which interferes with trypsin, one of the digestive enzymes.

While the milk is still warm, add 2 Tbsp. honey and 1 tsp. salt. Stir until dissolved. Pour into quart jars. Cover milk tightly and store in the refrigerator. Strain milk before use because a skin often forms on the surface.

Soybean Oil

Soybeans are rich in polyunsaturated oil, which is extracted for commercial use. Many commercial vegetable oils contain soybean oil. Soybean oil contains no cholesterol.

Processed soybean oil is light in color, has a mild flavor, and can be used as oil in any recipe. Soybean oil keeps best at refrigerator temperature after opening.

Soybean Mash

The mash or pulp is the solid material left after soybean milk has been prepared. Some protein is retained in the mash. Mash has a bland flavor and a rather coarse texture. Use it in combination with other foods for its nutritive value or as an extender in ground-meat dishes.

Mash must be heated thoroughly to eliminate the beany flavor and to prevent spoilage. Place mash in the top of a double boiler. Cook slowly over boiling water for about 1 hour. If mash becomes too dry, moisten it with a little soy milk or water. Stir occasionally during cooking. Add 1 tsp. salt. Cool and store in refrigerator.

One pound of beans, prepared for milk, will yield 1 quart of mash.

Soybean Curd

Soybean curd may be purchased fresh in many grocery stores and specialty markets. Fresh curd is purchased in squares called cakes.

To use fresh curd in recipes, cut the curd and let stand a few minutes. Drain off liquid before adding to recipe.

To store fresh bean curd, cover with water and store, tightly covered, in the refrigerator. Change the water daily. The curd will remain fresh several days.

Canned soybean curd is also available. Canned curd is darker in color and has a slightly different flavor and texture than fresh curd. Drain canned curd thoroughly before using.

Packaged instant bean curd powder is another form available. Prepare according to package directions. Cut and use it in the same way as fresh or canned bean curd.

Soy Soufflé

1 cup mashed soybeans*	4 egg yolks
1 Tbsp. parsley	4 egg whites
1 Tbsp. minced onion	
½ tsp. salt—if beans are seasoned use ¼ tsp. salt	

Mix beans and seasonings together with beaten yolks. Beat egg whites until stiff and fold gently into bean mixture. Pour into buttered or oiled 10″ × 6″ or 8″ × 8″ baking dish and bake in pan of hot water in moderate 350° oven until firm, about 30 minutes. Serve immediately with cheese or mushroom sauce. Serves 4.

*We keep 2 cup-cartons of cooked soybeans in the freezer. They're left over from stovetop beans or casserole beans. They come in handy for a recipe like this or soybean spread, etc. Be sure to allow for thawing time before using.

Soybean Supper

2 cups dry soybeans
4 cups water
3 tsp. salt
1 large grated carrot
1 medium chopped onion
1 Tbsp. soy oil
1 Tbsp. soy sauce
1 Tbsp. vegetable flakes
   (dried)

1 tsp. sweet basil
1 tsp. white or black
   pepper
1 tsp. paprika
1 cup V-8 (or tomato) juice
1 Tbsp. whole-wheat flour

Soak beans in 8 cups water overnight. *Drain.* In the morning, pour into crock pot and add 4 cups water and salt.
Plug in the crock pot and add the carrot, onion, oil, seasonings, and V-8 juice. Turn dial to high and cook for 7 to 10
hours. Just before serving, stir in flour. Makes 4-6 servings.
Serve with hot corn bread and green salad.

Soybean Spread

2 cups cooked soy beans
4 Tbsp. tomato sauce
2 Tbsp. chopped onion
2 Tbsp. chopped Ortega
   chiles

1 Tbsp. wheat germ
¼ tsp. salt
¼ tsp. pepper

Place all the ingredients into your blender and mix. With a
wooden spoon press down the mixture until all the beans
are pureed. Stop and start blender as needed to mix well.
If necessary add more liquid (not too much as this makes a
good sandwich spread). This is delicious stuffed in celery,
used as a dip for vegetables, used as a spread for open-
faced sandwiches topped with cheese and broiled, and on
whole-wheat crackers.

Molasses Softies
(no eggs or milk)

½ cup butter
½ cup corn oil
½ cup honey
½ cup molasses
1 tsp. vanilla
grated rind of 1 lemon
1 cup oat flour or grind
  oatmeal in blender

1 cup raw cashews, rolled
  fine in plastic bag
1 cup soy flour
2 cups whole-wheat pastry
  flour
1 tsp. salt

Cream butter and oil together. Add honey, molasses, vanilla, lemon rind, oat flour, and nuts. Stir together well. Measure flours and salt into large sifter. Sift together and add to molasses mixture with wooden spoon as batter is thick. Drop by spoonfuls onto oiled cookie sheet. Bake in 350° oven for about 12 minutes.

Soybean Quesadillas

2-3 cups cooked soybeans*
1 dozen flour tortillas
1 lb. Jack cheese, grated

1 lb. Longhorn cheese,
  grated

Mash beans with a fork or chop in blender and heat in saucepan. Place tortillas on baking sheet and spread with soybeans. Cover beans generously with mixed cheeses. Place under broiler and cook until bubbly. Serve immediately with a tossed green salad. Serve fresh pineapple for dessert.

*The cooked soybeans can be from any recipe in this book. I had on hand the crock-pot beans and used them the first time I made this recipe. They were delicious and moist.

Super Soy Fritters

2 eggs, beaten
1 Tbsp. soy sauce
3 Tbsp. minced onion
¼ tsp. paprika
¼ tsp. white pepper
1 cup brown rice, cooked
    with salt

1 cup rolled oats
2 cups cooked soybeans,
    mashed (any beans from
    other recipes in this
    book or canned
    soybeans)

In mixing bowl beat eggs and stir in all the other ingredients. Blend well. Shape into 4″ patties and bake on a hot, oiled skillet or griddle until golden brown, about 5 minutes on each side. Serves 4-6. For a complete menu serve a hot green vegetable and a fresh salad with fruits of the season.

Soy Yogurt

1 quart soy milk
¼ cup yogurt culture
    OR

1 cup plain yogurt made
    with pure lactobacillus
    bulgaricus culture
    (unsweetened and
    without fruit). This is
    available at specialty
    stores.

Heat soy milk to 115° in saucepan. Remove from heat and add culture. Pour into a sterile jar (or one that has gone through the dishwasher to make it sanitary). Cover with foil or cheesecloth or clean kitchen towel. Place jar in a warm place and allow to stand overnight or until thick. (A pilot light on the gas stove will work.) Chill and serve plain or topped with honey, fresh fruit, or unsweetened canned pineapple.

Baked Soybeans

3 cups dried soybeans (1 cup uncooked soybeans equals 3 cups cooked.)
1 medium onion
½ cup diced celery
2 bay leaves
2 tsp. salt
2 Tbsp. oil
¼ cup dark molasses
2 Tbsp. prepared mustard
2 Tbsp. Worcestershire sauce
1 lb. stewed tomatoes or fresh tomatoes
4 or 6 slices cooked bacon

Cover soy beans with 12 cups of water and bring to a boil for 2 minutes. Remove from heat and let stand for 1 hour. Refrigerate overnight and drain. Cover with 8 cups of water. Add the onion, celery, and seasonings. Bring to a boil in a covered pan, reduce heat to low and simmer for about 3 hours. Remove from heat. Measure out 2 cups of the cooked beans to be used in a soy spread. Pour remaining beans into a 2-qt. casserole and add molasses, mustard, and Worcestershire. Bake for 2 hours at 300°. Remove from oven and add tomatoes. Top with bacon and return to oven for another 30 minutes. Serves 6-8.

If you like, divide the beans into two 1-qt. casseroles; bake one and freeze one.

Beans-N-Rice Loaf

3 eggs
¼ cup minced onion
¼ cup minced celery
1 med. tomato, diced fine
1 tsp. salt
1 Tbsp. soy sauce
1 tsp. paprika
½ tsp. white pepper
¼ cup powdered milk
2 cups cooked brown rice
2 cups cooked soybeans, chopped

Beat eggs in mixing bowl and add onion, celery, tomato, and seasonings. Stir in milk. Mix in brown rice and beans blending well. Pat mixture into a buttered loaf pan and bake for 20-30 minutes in a 350° oven. Serves 4-6.

Vegetable Sausages

1 egg, beaten
3 tomatoes, peeled and
  pureed in blender
2 Tbsp. soy oil
½ cup fresh wheat germ

2 cups cooked soybeans,
  mashed
½ tsp. salt
¼ tsp. sage
½ cup peanuts, crushed

Beat egg in mixing bowl and stir in tomatoes, oil, wheat germ, beans, salt, sage, and peanuts. Blend well and shape into sausages. Roll sausages in more wheat germ and brown in butter and oil mixture. This is a complement to hot tomato soup. Serves 4.

CHAPTER SEVEN

A Potpourri of Healing and Delight

And God said, Behold, I have given you every herb bearing seed, which is upon the face of all the earth ... —Genesis 1:29

Our self-reliant forefathers knew more about simple, inexpensive health care than many educated people do today. They knew which herbal remedy to take for a cold, and how to fight infection resulting from disease or injury. Herbs played an important role in these home remedies.

People of yesteryear drank delicious beverages made from various herbs. Camomile tea, for example, contains substances which have a mildly calming or tranquilizing effect. One cup will not put you in a dream world as tranquilizers may do, but taken regularly, camomile tea will gradually make the drinker more relaxed and provide a tranquilizing effect that is harmless and inexpensive.

Many herbal medicine plants are as common as weeds in our gardens. In fact, some of them look like weeds! Early Americans used them as a contribution to their home landscape where they were valued for their fragrance, dye, culinary values, and healing properties.

Herbs help us to have fun with food. They provide fragrance, color, and beauty both inside and outside the house. The subject of herbs and their uses is too large for the scope of this chapter. We shall limit our discussion to herbs that heal and those that add flavor.

Take an herb to lunch

Mention the word "herb" to most people and they think of a gourmet kitchen where exotic menus are being prepared. Creative cooks use a variety of herbs to add just a touch of something special to meat, vegetables, broths, or brews of assorted types.

When restricted diets are prescribed, oregano can be used in place of salt and sweet cicely may stand in for sugar. Fresh herbs are to be preferred, but of course dried herbs in bottles serve well. Twice as many fresh herbs as dried herbs are needed in a given recipe, as a rule of thumb. You'll need your family's vote on the amount of herbs used until you determine their preferences.

The Rodale Herb Book, published in Emmaus, Pennsylvania, by Rodale Press, provides an exhaustive guide to a large assortment of herbs.[1]

Following is our list of the most popular culinary herbs arranged alphabetically. Some we use more than others, of course, and we are continually discovering uses for herbs. You will, too, as you experiment.

Allspice: Obtained from the dried, unripe berry of the allspice tree, allspice is used in seasoning game, poultry stuffings, and sausage mixtures. Allspice adds to the flavor of stews, sauces, and gravies. Small amounts of allspice are used for hot puddings, cakes, and fruit desserts.

Angelica: A hardy plant with a sweet taste used to decorate cakes and other desserts. A confection is made from the candied stem. Angelica serves well as a sweetener when mixed with sauces and can be cooked and eaten by itself.

Anise: This herb tastes and smells like licorice. Its leaves can be chopped and added to salads, cream sauces, and certain recipes for shellfish. When the plant produces seeds they can be used whole with sweet pickles, salad dressings, coffee cakes, and soups. The seeds can also be crushed and used for flavoring pastries. The oil of Anise is the base for licorice flavors. "Aniseed" is similar to "sweet cumin" in flavor and is used in making cakes, pastry, and confections.

Basil: A favorite with cooks, this "herb of love" has almost unlimited usages. Its most common use is with tomatoes—sprinkled over raw slices with an oil and vinegar salad dressing or put into tomato or spaghetti sauce. Basil finds its way into cheese and vegetable dishes, poultry and veal, and also into baked goods such as rolls and breads. It is a popular herb for French, Spanish, Italian, and Portuguese dishes.

Bay leaves: A penetrating herb, bay leaves complement cooked meats. An average-sized stew requires only half a leaf. Bay leaves enhance the flavor of tongue and corned beef. Soups and casseroles also enjoy a happy marriage with bay leaves.

Borage: With a taste akin to the cucumber's, borage is nicknamed the "herb of courage." It picks up the flavor of iced tea and fruit drinks, salads, and soups.

Bouquet garni: A group of herbs tied together for easy removal from the food.

Caraway: Few people have missed the seeds of caraway sprinkled on breads and pastries and their distinctive flavor. The herb can be added to the water for boiling potatoes or sprinkled over sauerkraut before it is cooked.

Caraway is delightful in potato salad, applesauce, or cheese. Caraway seeds rubbed into a pork loin can add a whole new dimension of flavor to the meat.

Cardamom: This is the prime ingredient in hot curry powders and sauces. Cardamom is a spice which one associates with orange flavor.

Chervil: Like parsley, but sweeter, chervil tastes a bit like anise. It serves well as a garnish for almost any dish or as a flavor inside the food. Chefs use it with corn or potato soup, salads, salad dressings, chicken, and fish. It is excellent for sauces and soups and is popular when used in cheese omelets.

Chili powder: A combination of several kinds of hot peppers, oregano, dried garlic, paprika, and cumin seed, which is used in preparing numerous dishes in Mexico.

Chives: Nearly everybody has been introduced to chives, the onion substitute. A low-calorie salad, sour cream, baked potatoes, and cottage cheese all receive chives well. Garlic (or Chinese) chives can be used just like the ordinary kind for distinctive, pleasant flavor.

Cinnamon: Cinnamon comes from dried inner bark of the cinnamon tree. It is important in making apple treats, and is also used in puddings, cakes, and sauces.

Cloves: Distinctive in aroma and having a hot, spicy flavor, cloves are excellent when added to pickles, pork, ham, spice cakes, gingerbread, and puddings.

Comfrey: The leaves of comfrey make a good salad; they can also be cooked like spinach. Young, tender leaves of this healthful herb are best.

Coriander: This herb is used like parsley. Its flavor is like a combination of sage and lemon. Its leaves yield vitamin C and taste good in curries, soups, and salads. Go easy; their flavor is pungent. The seeds of coriander are used in curry powder, pickling spices, and other spice mixtures. Ground coriander may be used to flavor cookies, rolls, custards, and pastries.

Cumin: This hot spice picks up Mexican-type foods and is used in curry and chili powder. Industry adds it to certain meats, pickles, cheese, and sausage. This spice is seasoning for Mexican, Far East, Oriental, and Indian cooking. It has a pronounced flavor.

Dandelions: To most people dandelions are pesky weeds to be pulled out of lawns and gardens. But their vitamin content makes them a nutritious source of food. The root makes an edible vegetable; the plant, before it blooms, has edible leaves like spinach that are good in salads. Pennsylvania Dutch people use it as a diuretic.

Dill: The most common companion of dill seed is pickles. The annual plant is easily grown and is harvested as dillweed before the seed head forms. Dill seed is added to relishes, sour cream, butter and fish sauces, spiced beets, and numerous other foods.

Egyptian onions: "Top Onions" or "separators" are other names for the Egyptian onion. It tastes like a mild onion and can be pickled for soups and stews and other dishes in which onion flavor is desired.

Fennel: Fennel seeds are good as flavor enhancers in bread, cakes, pastries, soups, stews, sweet pickles, fish, and sauerkraut. Fish sauces and chicken and egg dishes taste good when seasoned with fresh fennel greens. Fennel in salmon or mackerel helps to reduce the oiliness. "Finocchio" is a variety of fennel. It grows like celery and can be eaten raw or boiled as a vegetable. Italians and Mediterranean French are especially fond of this herb.

Ginger: Ginger originated in southern China and was one of the first Oriental spices. It enhances the flavor of steaks and chops. Applesauces, stewed fruits, and chutneys are better tasting because of ginger.

Horehound: Used mostly as a tea, horehound can help to

chase sore throats, colds, and coughs. It is also used to make horehound candy.

Horseradish: A large root, horseradish has a sharp, stinging sort of taste. The root, peeled and ground, can be mixed with vinegar and served with beef and other meats. It is loaded with vitamin C. Served with raw oysters and smoked tongue, it adds zip and interest. A drop on a peanut butter cracker makes a delicious hors d'oeuvre. Occasionally the spring shoots of horseradish are cooked as greens.

Lemon balm: "A tea smelling like lemon" best describes this herb. Lemon balm dresses up soups, stews, custards, puddings, or baked goods. Occasionally it can be used successfully in salad dressings and in iced tea and fruit drinks.

Mace: Although an expensive spice, mace is still a popular seasoning for cakes, puddings, fish, and shellfish, cauliflower, and carrots.

Marjoram: The taste of sweet marjoram is often confused with oregano because the two have resemblances in appearance and taste. Marjoram, however, is sweeter and milder than oregano. Marjoram, added to ordinary garden vegetables, provides a new dimension of flavor. Serve it with beef dishes (meat loaf, stew, meat sauce) or with omelets, scrambled eggs, gravies, sauces, and poultry stuffings. Marjoram tastes good sprinkled on green salad, bean dishes, and tomatoes.

Mint: A variety of mints (orange, lemon balm, spearmint, peppermint) go well with iced tea. Leaves from mint plants are tasty on peas, carrots, potatoes, and fish. Lamb is not complete without a dash of mint sauce. Added to a fruit cup it garnishes the dish beautifully.

Nasturtium leaves: Leaves from a tender young nasturtium plant add a peppery zip to soups and salads. In the winter they can be used dried. The seed pods of the nasturtium plant can be harvested like capers. The flowers, too, are interesting when served as a salad's garnish.

Nutmeg: A very delicate and aromatic tropical fruit, nutmeg serves to enhance many foods. A membrane covering the kernel provides mace, another spice.

Oregano: Pizza pies have made oregano famous in America. The herb is also added to spaghetti, homemade tomato sauce, and pureed tomatoes. Oregano adds a delightful flavor to stews, gravies, salads, and tomato juice. It adds zest to a variety of bland vegetables like squash.

Paprika: Color and flavor are the contributions of paprika to many French, Spanish, and Hungarian recipes. It is the primary ingredient of the Hungarian national dish—gulyas. Poultry and veal are improved with paprika.

Parsley: Vitamin C in this rough little green? Yes, although more often than not parsley is used to garnish foods and tossed aside as a bitter herb. Add pieces of it to boiled and buttered potatoes, fish, meats, and vegetables. Omelets taste better and look better with bits of parsley included. Sprigs of it immersed in a soup while it is being stewed can add flavor. Parsley is often used with bay leaf and thyme for *bouquet garni.*

Pepper: Probably the most widely used of all spices, pepper is available in black, red, or white varieties.

Rosemary: The wide-ranging uses of this versatile herb spread from breads to meats to jams to desserts. Rosemary leaves can be rubbed into such meat as lamb, duck, chicken, or pork before roasting. Rosemary leaves add a touch of sweetness to fruit cups, punches, and marinating sauces. Small boiled potatoes fried with rosemary result in a tasty, crunchy meal. Use sparingly.

Rue: Just a touch of rue goes well in salads or traditionally on pumpernickel bread. Butter the bread and sprinkle rue over it for a tasty, different bit of culinary delight.

Saffron: Italians, French, and Spaniards all use saffron to give food that extra zip. It is used in soups, in rice dishes, and sometimes in baking.

Sage: Poultry stuffing tastes that way because of sage leaves to which we've grown accustomed. Sausage, liver, fish, and cheese also contain sage quite often. Sometimes it's good with pickles and onions.

Savory: Called "Bohnenkraut" in Germany, savory picks up flavor in beans and other legumes. Summer savory grows only in the summer; winter savory grows into part of the cold season. Both types flavor hot or cold bean dishes, lentils, meats, or poultry stuffing delightfully. Potato salad can make good use of the young shoots of savory.

Sorrel (French): French sorrel tastes good in soups and salads. Tender young sorrel leaves can be mixed with lettuce for a salad; older leaves taste sour and should be submerged in soup. With raisins and honey they combine to make a dessert something like rhubarb.

Sweet cicely: Tasting something like anise, sweet cicely can replace a sweetener in fruit pies, coffee cakes, cooked fruits, salads, and salad dressings. Fish and carrots taste good with sweet cicely added. You can eat its roots raw or boiled. The seeds of sweet cicely taste like licorice candy.

Tarragon: Perhaps one of the best known among herbs, tarragon is used in seafood and chicken dishes. It helps remove fishy taste from seafood. Tarragon is also helpful in flavoring leafy salads, most vegetables, and cream sauces.

Thyme: This herb enhances the flavor of soups, fish chowders, poultry, and lamb. Try using lemon thyme in chicken dressing for an interesting flavor. Oregano thyme can be substituted for oregano; caraway thyme can replace caraway; upright thymes serve best in cooking. Sprinkle the herb on carrots, beef and lamb stews, chicken and fish dishes. Thyme in grape, elderberry, and apple jellies complement lamb dishes.

A Rose by Any Other Name

Few moments in life are more pleasurable than a midday break for a pot of herbal tea. Following our reading of C. S. Lewis's *Chronicles of Narnia,* a seven-volume series, to our boys at the supper table one winter, our youngsters began sharing our tea breaks. Like Lucy, Peter, Edmund, et al, they enjoyed their experience with tea and cookies—our own pastries concocted from healthful recipes contained in another part of this book.

But herbs do more than just flavor, garnish, and make plain foods memorable. Many have blooms which can be used creatively in cooking. Some flowers from herbs also provide color accents in landscaping and interior decorating, and splashes of artistic charm for salads and pastries.

Among the herbal blooms you can use are the following, listed in alphabetical order:

Calendula flowers: Blooms from this plant make rich, golden colors for butter, cheese, sauces, soups, and stews. When saffron is unavailable, calendula flowers are a fine substitute. The calendula colors and flavors tea as well as foods.

Chives: Smelling strong but looking sweet is the pretty flower of chives which garnishes potato or macaroni salads and makes any meal look festive and appetizing.

Marigolds: As their name would suggest, marigolds color any spread with a golden glow. When used as a flavor booster they add a robust touch to rice, soups, and stews.

Nasturtiums: Coming on strong like pepper, the blossom of the nasturtium can be sprinkled on salads or used whole to garnish fruit plates. Some chefs mince the blossoms and blend them with butter.

Rose petals: Cooks have used rose petals for many years and for a variety of reasons. They've made rose water, rose syrup, and rose petal jam. Rose petals used in fruit punches or to decorate pastries can add appeal to a meal. Ask for "tea roses" when you shop, but remember to cut off the white edge of each petal. Otherwise, your herb will add a tinge of bitterness to the food.

Safflower: The superb oil that the seed head of safflower yields is becoming increasingly popular. Safflower's petals can be used as standins to provide color for butter, rice, chicken gravy, or stew.

Saffron crocus: That golden coloring you see in recipes (as if an abundant supply of eggs were included) may come from this autumn-blooming crocus. Just a pinch of saffron will go a long way in flavoring and coloring butter, cheese, rice, noodles, chicken gravies, soups, and pastries.

Violets: Roses are red, violets are blue. They are also delicious in violet syrup, jams, and jellies. Candied violets, an extraordinary conversation piece for any table, can be used as a condiment or a cake decoration.

'Doctor Herb'

Herbs are used as accents in a landscape, as garnishings for a dish, as pleasing taste enhancers, and as teas. But there is yet another way to use herbs—as handy first-aid assistants in cases of mild disorders.

Burns

A poultice of mint leaves can assuage a searing burn when other medicine is unavailable.

Corns

Apply lemon juice or a fresh slice of garlic on a corn. Either substance should be covered with a bandage.

Headache

If a headache is caused by a chill, brew a hot cup of thyme tea for relief.

Hoarse throat

A gargle of sage and vinegar is helpful.

Indigestion

Fennel tea is mild and pleasant when indigestion brings discomfort.

Stiff joints

Pour boiling water over pine cones. When lukewarm, water can be used to bathe the joints or as a massage with corn oil, olive oil, or sunflower oil.

Nervousness

A pot of camomile or sage tea is calming. Beetroot juice is said also to be tranquilizing.

Vomiting

Take either lemon juice or apple cider vinegar in water after vomiting. This is to restore the acid balance in the stomach.

THINGS TO DO

1. Be adventuresome and grow your own herbs in pots in your kitchen.

2. Think of flowering herbs to garnish dishes.

3. Learn to enjoy herbal teas instead of harmful caffeine drinks.

4. Beautify your landscape design with herbal bushes.

5. Look to herbs for first-aid in uncomplicated cases of discomfort.

Beverly's Chicken Parisian

1 chicken (fryer, cut up)
1 cup vegetable oil
1 cup flour
Rice mixture:
2½ cups chicken stock (or 2 chicken bouillon cubes in same amount of water)
1 cup Uncle Ben's long grain raw rice

1 clove garlic, minced
1 cup onions, minced
2 tsp. salt
¼ tsp. black pepper
¼ tsp. thyme
⅛ tsp. marjoram
1 9-oz. pkg. frozen green beans

Rinse chicken; pat dry with paper towel; salt and pepper each piece. Pour flour into a paper bag and shake each piece of chicken in the bag to coat with flour. Brown the chicken in the hot oil. Drain on paper towel. In a 9″ x 13″ baking pan prepare the rice mixture. Mix stock, rice, and seasonings together and break up the frozen beans in the hot mixture. Place browned chicken on top and cover with foil. Bake for 1 hour in 350° oven. Serve on large platter with rice in center and garnished with slivered almonds. This may also be baked for three hours at 225°. This is handy for churchgoers on Sunday morning.

Herbed Fish Steaks

1 stick butter
¼ tsp. sweet basil
¼ tsp. marjoram
¼ tsp. tarragon
1 Tbsp. chives
1 Tbsp. minced parsley
1 tsp. garlic

½ cup onion, chopped
3 Tbsp. lemon juice
2 lbs. fresh fish (cod, haddock, halibut, or salmon)
1 cup bread crumbs, rolled fine

Soften butter to room temperature and mix in all the herbs and salt. If possible, make this the day before so herbs can blend and penetrate the butter. Melt herbed butter and add onion. Sauté gently until onions are tender. Add lemon juice and set aside. Arrange fish in a shallow baking pan or dish. Spoon half the herbed butter over the steaks. Pour remaining butter over the bread crumbs and blend. Cover steaks with this mixture and bake in 400° hot oven for 20-25 minutes. Serves 4-6. Plan to serve fresh string beans, sliced tomatoes, and baked potatoes.

Herbed Brown Rice

1 cup brown rice
2⅔ cups water
1 tsp. salt
1 Tbsp. soy oil
¼ tsp. thyme
¼ tsp. marjoram

¼ cup green onion, sliced diagonally
⅓ cup sliced almonds with skin on
2 Tbsp. soy oil

Bring water to a rolling boil, add salt, herbs, oil, and rice. Reduce heat to low and simmer for 40-50 minutes. (Increase cooking time in high altitude.)

Sauté onions and nuts in oil. When rice is tender and all the water is absorbed, add the onions and nuts. Blend and serve piping hot. Serves 5-6.

Grandma Bechtel's Carrot Relish

10 cups carrots
10 cups cucumbers;
  remove seeds
5 cups red and green
  peppers
2 cups onion
3½ cups sugar (adapt for
  your needs with honey
  or artificial sweetener)

2 cups water
3 cups cider vinegar
2 Tbsp. salt
2 Tbsp. celery seed
1 Tbsp. dry mustard
4 Tbsp. flour
1 tsp. turmeric

Chop all the vegetables into small pieces. Cook carrots until almost tender and add the other vegetables. Combine sugar, water, salt, vinegar, and celery seed and pour over vegetables. Simmer slowly for several minutes. With a small amount of water make a smooth paste with the flour, mustard, and turmeric. Stir into simmering vegetables and boil for 5 minutes. Pour into hot sterile jars. Seal. Makes 10 pints.

Herb Tea Suggestions

Alfalfa mint, peppermint,
  raspberry leaf, papaya
  leaf, sassafras bark,
  fennel seed, mistletoe,
  camomile.

CHAPTER EIGHT

Escape from Allergies

Weep no more my lady, O weep no more today.
—Stephen Collins Foster,
"My Old Kentucky Home, Good Night"

Allergies are diseases caused by substances which are harmful only to people who are sensitive to them. Often they surface in people who endure long periods of stress.

At the top of the list among offenders are milk, wheat, and eggs. Material which causes an allergic reaction is called an allergen. As many as six out of ten people have shown some allergic reaction at some time during their lives. Children can inherit tendencies toward allergies but not an allergy itself.

A medical explanation showing how allergies begin states that they result when an allergen combines with a specific body protein called an antibody. The combination causes cells to release histamine into the bloodstream and tissues. Histamine is a substance normally found in the cells of the body. As long as it remains in the cells, it does no

167

harm. But when too much histamine is released from the cells it affects the blood vessels and causes the tissues around them to swell. Excessive histamine in different parts of the body produces different kinds of allergic symptoms.

In 1965 a judge in Oklahoma City wrote a book on his deliverance from allergies which became almost instantly a pacesetter in the field. Judge Tom R. Blaine linked allergic reaction to nutrition and successfully proved that many people who suffer from allergies are hypoglycemic. He discovered that lazy adrenal glands and an unhealthy endocrine system are the real culprits in allergies.

"Doctors tell us we are as old as our arteries," Judge Blaine wrote, "but I say we are as well as our endocrines. It is my belief, based on my experience, that the greatest medical discovery of this age, as far as allergy sufferers are concerned, is that weak and diseased adrenal glands (even if inherited) can be made into healthy adrenals by medication and by a diet which does not place too much strain on them."[1]

People who suffer from allergies tend also to be nervous types, often depressed and irritable. But these people also seem to be a cut above the norm in terms of achievement. Surveys show that they have relatively higher intelligence than other people. They are usually meticulous in their work habits, driving themselves to exhaustion. They don't know how to relax, don't pursue hobbies that are personally satisfying, and have married their work.

Allergics complain to their doctors that they are tired, can't sleep, and feel pessimistic about life, all the while driving hard to accomplish their goals.

Fatigue is so constant a companion to an allergic that he is usually too tired to exercise as he knows he should. Allergy patients pay more for health treatments, yet they often feel unwelcome in the doctor's office.

Point of order

Judge Blaine discovered that tired and diseased adrenal glands can become healthy organs by stimulating the glands with medication and observing a strict diet high in proteins and without any processed commercial sugar. Many hypoglycemics also suffer from allergies. In these cases the pancreas is overstimulated by sugar and excretes too much insulin. This burns up the sugar quickly, leaving the victim with low blood sugar, feelings of depression, fatigue, and low stamina.

In his practice as a trial judge, author Blaine observed that about 50 percent of his court cases were married people seeking a divorce from their spouses. A typical complaint from a wife was that her husband was always tired and unable to hold a job. The wife, who was forced to get a job to provide for the family, would conclude bitterly that if she could shed her mate she would have one less mouth to feed.

From husbands seeking divorces from wives, Judge Blaine heard a similar complaint. The wife had become a sloppy housekeeper, ate too much, spent too much time in bed, and lost her zest for living. Doctors in both cases could usually find nothing organically wrong, so the spouse had to conclude that the mate was lazy.

In such cases Judge Blaine recommended that the couple's physician arrange for a six-hour glucose tolerance test to determine whether the offending party were suffering from low blood sugar. The judge found that when clients tending toward hypoglycemia would follow a high protein, sugarless diet for an endocrine gland condition, the depression and fatigue would often disappear. The hapless victim often dramatically became a "new person." Often the divorce proceedings were dropped.

Allergy and aggression

Physical violence in children has been traced directly to allergic reactions. *Psychology Today* stated in its July 1975 issue: "For an allergic person, eating may lead to beating, biting and battle. While a person who is allergic to pollen suffers a stuffy nose, a person allergic to chocolate or bananas may pass out [give other people] bloody noses."

Author K. E. Moyer, Professor of Psychology at Carnegie-Mellon University, Pittsburgh, found that children who suffered severe reactions to food or medicine or pollens could be dramatically delivered from the scourge. He calls his descriptions of reactions among allergics "a veritable thesaurus of irritability." Victims are "impulsive, combative, unruly, perverse, and quarrelsome."

A girl ten years old suffered an asthma attack when exposed to alcohol. She was totally amnesiac during the period of her attack, with moods ranging from silliness to withdrawal. Several times she grew angry and aggressive. She tried to bite her mother, whom she did not recognize.

Another case described a nine-year-old boy who reacted so violently to wheat that he awakened from a nightmare completely disoriented. He could not say where he was, who he was, or who his parents were. The child beat his head repeatedly against the wall and screamed uncontrollably.

Another boy studied was plagued with temper tantrums. Physicians termed him "aphasic" because his speech was developed poorly. He was too uncontrollable to sit for an IQ examination.

Allergy tests on the boy showed strong reactions to yeast, chocolate, and milk. An electroencephalogram displayed fourteen-per-second "spikes," large amounts of sharp activity in the motor leads, temporal single polyphasic sharp waves and a long run of sharp waves in the right temporal area.

A diet free of milk, chocolate, and cola drinks began at once to offer relief. His electroencephalogram seven and a half months later was normal. Six months later he was learning better and his behavior had greatly improved. The offending foods were administered again as a test, resulting in the same reactions.

Dr. Moyer concluded in his study that many more people suffer from symptoms of allergy (fatigue, irritability, pallor, nasal congestion, and other emotional symptoms of a great variety) than a general reading of allergy texts would indicate. How many erratic, nervous, and mentally disabled people could have been helped out of their maladies through diet? The idea is spurring the researchers on.

"Unless we continue the search for a means of control," Dr. Moyer concludes, "our increasing technological capability to translate violence into death may answer the questions for us."

The Chemical Scourge

Read the label!

After observing the nutritional trinity of proper *food*, *exercise*, and *rest*, there is a fourth matter that may save your life: Avoid eating too many deadly chemicals which are proliferating in the foods we eat.

A smattering of random newspaper headlines provides an ominous warning: "Americans Eat Fungicide-Treated Lemons Banned in Japan," "Hundreds of Thousands of Cancer-Causing Chemicals Out of Control Threaten Consumers," "Lead Poisoning Reexamined," "Technologists Seek Longest Shelf Life," "Sodium Nitrite Produces Brain

Changes," "Government Approving Thousands of Food Additives That Threaten Your Health...," etc.

One autumn day the news media announced that Red Dye No. 2 was found to be carcinogenic. The dye was ordered off the market, but the food processing plants complained that they had no workable substitute. The dye remained on the market for many months in soft drinks, fruit drinks, cereals, desserts, diet desserts, candy, and miscellaneous items.

The dye, produced from beetles' eggs imported from Central America, was used in Fanta grape, strawberry, red creme soda, and cherry soft drinks. It was also used in Tang, Kool-Aid, Hi-C grape, Wyler's low-calorie fruit drink mixes, Royal gelatins, Life Savers in raspberry, grape, and cherry flavors, Open-Pit barbecue sauce, and certain soups. Lipstick, strawberry ice cream, and many other commodities were contaminated by Red Dye No. 2. Unfortunately, workable substitutes have not been found for all items, so the dye is still a part of the food we eat.

Dr. Herbert Ley, Jr., shortly after he was relieved of his job as Commissioner of the Food and Drug Administration, stated, "The thing that bugs me is that the people think the FDA is protecting them. It isn't. What the FDA is doing and what the public thinks it's doing are as different as day and night." His remarks were quoted by Jaqueline Verrett and Jean Carper in *Eating May Be Hazardous to Your Health* (Anchor Books, N.Y., 1975).

The ranks of those against food additives has its share of fanatics and exaggerators, but there is logic behind their program. Many thoughtful scientists are frankly worried about the vast increases of strange new chemicals dumped into human food to preserve shelf life, tickle the palate, and delight the eye.

There are at present more than 1,000 chemicals in our

foods that have never been tested for their potentialities of causing cancer, genetic damage, or birth defects, according to veteran researcher Beatrice Trum Hunter in her book, *Food Additives and Your Health* (Keats Publishing, New Canaan, Conn., 1972).

"The public *wrongly* assumes that all chemicals contained in foods (and drugs) have been tested for safety and effectiveness," says Mrs. Hunter. "Unfortunately, this is not true. Hundreds of chemicals on a list of substances 'Generally Recognized as Safe' known as the GRAS list, and other substances routinely used by the food industry have never been fully tested for possible harmful effects."

If the 1958 Federal Food Additive Amendment had been vigorously enforced, Mrs. Hunter declared in her book, "a majority of the chemical additives on the GRAS list would probably have been excluded."

Even though the FDA is charged with policing the processing of food, manufacturers, with the FDA's agreement, have kept for themselves the right to determine whether or not a food additive is safe. Food processors have not been forced to file a petition for using an additive or even to inform the FDA of its planned use. Even when other sources tag a chemical unsafe, the FDA has been slow to enforce the law, failing to act quickly and decisively.

Once a food additive makes it to the GRAS list, it is exempt from the "additive" label. At that point it is not subject to regulations governing food additives. To remove it, the FDA must first prove its harmfulness. A better policy would be to pre-test every food additive before it is marketed.

An expert in the study of food additives declared that 485 compounds out of several thousand currently in use do not have to be listed on the labels! It is known that food additives can have a devastating effect on the hyperkinetic child, aggravating his unstable condition.

An observer in Washington stated that if thalidomide had not produced such grotesque physical shapes in newborn babies, and only genetic deficiencies, it would "still be dispensed like aspirin."

The average American consumes five pounds of chemical additives each year. The food in your market basket contains artificial flavor enhancers, preservatives, antioxidants, emulsifiers, stabilizers, thickeners, acidulants, colors, bleaching, maturing agents, humectants (to keep food moist), anticaking agents, firming agents, clarifying agents, curing agents, foaming agents, foam inhibitors, and nonnutritive sweeteners.

For example, Americans consume 800 million gallons of ice cream each year. Most give little thought to the ingredients, not knowing they are digesting a small chemical laboratory. Ice cream manufacturers are not required to label these additives which include: *Piperonal,* used instead of vanilla. This is a chemical used to kill lice. *Aldehyde C17,* a flavor for cherry ice cream. It is an inflammable liquid used also in anilene dyes, plastic, and rubber. *Diethyl glucol,* an inexpensive chemical used as an emulsifier in place of eggs. Diethyl glucol is the same substance used in antifreeze and in paint removers. *Ethyl acetate* gives ice cream a pineapple flavor. It's a chemical used also to clean leather and textiles. Its vapors have caused chronic lung, liver, and heart damage. *Butyraldehyde* gives ice cream a nut flavor. It is also used in rubber cement. *Amyl acetate* provides a banana flavor, and is a chemical also used as an oil paint solvent. *Benzyl acetate* in ice cream gives it a strawberry flavor. It is a nitrate solvent.

Come and get it, folks! The fresh, tangy flavor of butylated hydroxytoluene ... the home-cooked goodness of calcium disodium EDTA ... the satisfying richness of sodium carboxymethylcellulose ....

THINGS TO DO

1. Minimize allergy symptoms by avoiding stressful situations.

2. Depression can be a warning signal of allergic reaction to foods or chemicals. See a specialist.

3. Experiment continually by eliminating foods suspected of producing undesirable reactions.

4. Allergic reactions can stem from glandular dysfunction. See an endocrinologist for tests if an allergen cannot be identified.

5. Enjoy the following wheat-free, chocolate-free, and sugar-free recipes.

Carob

The curious "chocolate" called "St. John's Bread," "honey locust," and other colorful names, allows you to have your cake and eat it too.

This brown powder used as the basis for luscious desserts is made from finely ground pods taken off budding trees. The pods are found on a tree similar in appearance to an apple tree. It grows profusely as a dark evergreen tree in the Mediterranean regions. Some say John the Baptist ate it to survive in the wilderness.

Carob powder is rich in potassium, calcium, and phosphorus. It contains, in smaller amounts, magnesium, silicon, and iron. Because of its rich mineral content it is considered a bowel conditioner. Its appearance resembles cocoa. It is high in vitamin A and niacin with trace amounts of B_1 and B_2.

Carob is rich in natural sugars, low in starch, low in fat (only 2 percent fat compared with 52 percent in chocolate). It is delicious in brownies, hot drinks, cakes, and healthful confections. The flavor is different from chocolate, but the palate can be educated to enjoy it with relish. We tried it out on some teen-agers and they decided it was just as good as cocoa. It is so mild it can even be fed to small children, providing extra calcium and phosphorus for teeth and bones.

If your market doesn't stock carob, ask your grocer to order it for you. As more and more cooks eliminate chocolate from their cooking, the demand for a natural substitute will grow. Remember, chocolate is high in saturated fat and should not be allowed in the diet of anyone with heart disease, high blood pressure, or diabetes.

"Chocolate," said our doctor, "is to be sold, not eaten."

That made it tough for us chocolate lovers until we discovered carob. Carob can be used as a direct replacement for cocoa. In recipes calling for cocoa, use an equal amount of carob powder. In recipes calling for chocolate, use 3 Tbsp. carob powder plus 1 Tbsp. water to equal one square of chocolate.

Carob Ice Cream Pie

2 cups granola (see page 251)
2 Tbsp. butter
1 Tbsp. carob
2 Tbsp. water
1 large ripe banana

1 quart carob ice cream, made with honey
Topping:
1 cup whipping cream
1 Tbsp. honey
1 tsp. carob powder

Melt butter and add carob and water, mixing well over low heat. Pour over granola and toss to mix. Spread mixture in a buttered 9″ pie plate. Chill. Slice banana over crust. Soften ice cream slightly and spread over bananas, pressing down evenly with back of spoon. Whip cream and add honey and carob. Swirl over ice cream and freeze until firm. Remove from freezer 15 minutes before cutting. Serves 6-8.

Carob Brownies

½ cup sifted rice flour
½ cup sifted oat flour
½ cup sifted carob powder
½ tsp. baking powder
¼ tsp. salt
2 egg yolks

¾ cup honey or molasses
⅓ cup safflower oil or
  other vegetable oil
2 tsp. vanilla
2 egg whites

Place all dry ingredients in a large sifter and sift into a mixing bowl. Beat egg yolks and add honey, oil, and vanilla, mixing well. Pour over dry ingredients and blend completely. Beat egg whites until stiff, and gently fold into the carob batter. Pour into 10″ × 6″ buttered pan. If glass, bake at 325°, or otherwise at 350° for 30 minutes.

Hot "Chocolate"
(Actually delicious, nutritious carob)

¼ cup carob powder
½ cup water
4 cups milk (nonfat is fine)
⅛ tsp. or pinch of salt

¼ cup honey (or increase
  to taste)
1 tsp. vanilla

Mix powder and water in saucepan and bring to a simmer. Add milk and salt and heat. Watch closely so it doesn't boil. Stir honey and vanilla into carob milk, blending well. Serve immediately. If it must wait, cover and be sure to use a flat utensil to stir up the carob, because it tends to settle on the bottom.

Children relish this drink. It's the perfect answer for the youngster who loves hot chocolate but is allergic to it or can't tolerate refined sugar. This drink is actually healthful. The young people who sampled it for me decided it was better than the traditional hot chocolate. It is a favorite with skiers and snowmobilers.

Snack suggestion: Serve with sesame seed bars and cold, crisp apples.

Carob Fudge Sauce

½ cup carob powder   ⅓ cup butter
½ cup honey   1 tsp. vanilla
⅔ cup evaporated milk

Mix carob, honey, and milk together. Cook over medium heat, stirring constantly until syrup comes to a boil. Boil for one minute while stirring. Remove from heat. Add butter and vanilla. Beat well.

This is a delicious sauce and can also be used in hot or cold milk.

Protein-Packed Cookie Snack

½ cup softened butter   1 Tbsp. baking powder
½ cup vegetable oil   ⅓ cup bran flakes
1½ cups honey   ⅓ cup raw wheat germ
4 beaten eggs   1 cup crushed pecans (put
1 Tbsp. vanilla   in plastic bag and crush
½ cup soy flour   with rolling pin—brings
2 cups whole-wheat flour*   out flavor more than
½ cup powdered skim   chopping)
    milk   1 cup sesame seeds
¼ or ½ cup carob powder   1½ cups currants or dates
¾ tsp. salt

Beat first five ingredients together until blended. Measure next six items into large sifter and sift into above mixture. Stir until ingredients are well mixed. Add last five ingredients and stir until all are combined. Batter will be sticky. You may add other nuts or sunflower seeds or whatever variety you have. Be creative. Bake for 10 minutes in 325° oven. Sesame seeds brown quickly, so watch carefully. Happy eating!

*If allergic to wheat, use oat flour, barley flour, or rice flour. Eliminate bran and add oatmeal or more nuts. Some people allergic to wheat can tolerate fresh wheat germ—use your own judgment.

Apricot-Pineapple Bread

1 cup dried apricots
1¾ cup water
2 cups oat flour
1¼ cup rice flour
¼ cup soy flour
½ cup nonfat dry milk
3 tsp. baking powder
1 tsp. salt

3 eggs, beaten
1 cup honey
¼ cup vegetable oil
remaining liquid from
  apricots
½ cup crushed pineapple
  with some juice
chopped apricots

In saucepan cover apricots with water and simmer fruit until it is tender but still has body. Cool. Sift all dry ingredients into mixing bowl. Beat eggs well and add honey, oil, and apricot liquid. Stir in crushed pineapple and blend well. Add this to the dry ingredients and combine until moistened. Now add the chopped apricots, folding in and distributing throughout the batter. Butter two 3½″ × 7½″ loaf pans and divide the batter between them. Bake in a moderate oven 350° for approximately 30 minutes. Watch carefully, as soy flour browns quickly. If you use glass pans, reduce heat to 325°.

Strawberry Ice Cream

2 cups strawberries,
  washed
½ cup powdered milk
½ cup honey

2 cups plain yogurt
1 cup whipping cream
1 tsp. vanilla

Place berries and powdered milk in blender and whiz in honey. Pour into mixing bowl and *fold* in yogurt. Cover with foil and partially freeze. Remove and whip with egg beaters. Whip cream with vanilla, using an egg beater or electric mixer.* Fold whipped cream into strawberries and freeze.
*Cream doesn't whip well in blender.

New Mexico Corn Bread

2 eggs	¼ cup soy flour
¾ cup milk	1 tsp. baking powder
⅓ cup safflower oil	2 cups grated longhorn
1 cup cream style corn	cheese
1 cup cornmeal	1 4-oz. can diced green
1 tsp. salt	chiles

Beat eggs and add all the other ingredients in the order given, mixing with a wooden spoon. Pour batter into an oiled 10″ × 6″ pan. Bake in hot oven 400° for 40-45 minutes. If using a glass pan, reduce temperature and bake for approximately 35 minutes. This is a heavy, moist cornbread unlike the cake type. Some even like it cold, or it can be warmed successfully.

Our friend and veteran nutritionist, Lorraine Austin (forced into wheat-free customized cooking for needs among her children), shares this favorite main dish. She serves this with a gargantuan tossed green salad for a complete meal.

Christmas Wreath Cookies

1 stick butter	green food coloring
30 marshmallows	5 cups cornflakes
¼ cup pecans, crushed in plastic bag	

Place butter and marshmallows in top of double boiler. Melt over moderate heat, stirring as needed. Add pecans. Remove from heat and stir in enough food coloring to make a bright color. Pour over cornflakes, mixing well.

Dip hands in cold water and form mixture into 2″ wreaths. Press three cinnamon candies across the top to resemble holly berries. Place wreaths on cookie sheet covered with wax paper. Place wax paper on top of cookies and allow to stand overnight until well set.

Christmas Marmalade

1 lemon
1 orange
1 grapefruit

1 cup honey
1 Tbsp. butter

Peel and slice the fruits very thin. Place in stainless steel or glass container and cover with 1½ quarts cold water. Cover and allow to stand for 2 days in a cool place. Pour into kettle and add honey. Bring to a boil and simmer for 1 hour. Stir often. Add 1 Tbsp. butter and cool. Pour into sanitary jars and store in refrigerator.

Homemade Graham Crackers
(Sugarless)

2 cups whole-wheat
  graham flour
1 cup unbleached flour
½ tsp. salt
1 tsp. ground coriander
½ tsp. ground cinnamon

½ cup raw bran flakes
1 Tbsp. arrowroot powder
½ cup vegetable oil
½ cup milk
⅓ cup honey
¼ cup molasses

In a large sifter, sift flours, salt, and spices together. Add bran flakes and arrowroot. Stir in oil and blend well. Mix milk, honey, and molasses together and pour over flour mixture. Gather into a ball and knead slightly. Spread onto floured board and roll out thin. Cut into squares, pierce with a fork, and bake in 275° oven for 25 minutes.

Berry Blintzes

Pancakes:
3 eggs
2 cups milk
½ tsp. salt
1 cup oat flour
2 Tbsp. melted butter
1 tsp. vanilla
Filling:
1 cup cottage cheese
1 3-oz. pkg. cream cheese,
   softened

1 Tbsp. lemon rind
2 Tbsp. lemon juice
2 Tbsp. honey
¼ tsp. vanilla
Topping:
2 pkgs. frozen
   strawberries or 2 boxes
   fresh strawberries

Beat eggs and add milk, salt, and flour. Beat together well. Add butter. Spoon 2 Tbsp. batter onto lightly greased griddle or a small skillet. Bake until small bubbles appear; then loosen edges gently, turn and bake.

Whip cheeses and flavorings together until creamy. Spoon about 2 Tbsp. onto each pancake. Roll up and place in baking dish. Heat in 400° oven for 10 minutes. Makes 15-20. These may be made the night before and stored in refrigerator. Cover.

Thaw berries and heat through without cooking. If berries are frozen, add 1 Tbsp. lemon juice—if fresh, omit lemon juice and sweeten only if necessary. Spoon over hot blintzes and serve.

Brunch Menu:
   Fresh fruit cup of oranges and bananas
   Berry blintzes
   Ham slice
   Milk and hot drink

Sesame Seed Waffles
(preheat waffle iron)

2 cups flour (Oat, barley, or rice. If not allergic to wheat use whole wheat.)
¼ cup soy flour
4 tsp. baking powder
1 tsp. salt
6 egg yolks
1⅓ cups milk
¼ cup soy oil (or other vegetable oil)
6 egg whites
2 tsp. vanilla
sesame seeds
melted butter
warm honey or pure maple syrup

Sift flour into measuring cups. Pour flour into larger sifter and add baking powder and salt. Sift into large mixing bowl. In small mixing bowl beat egg yolks, add milk and oil. Combine with dry ingredients, blending until well absorbed. Beat egg whites until stiff but not dry. Fold into mixture with a light touch. Add vanilla. Spoon batter onto preheated waffle iron and sprinkle with one teaspoon sesame seeds. Serve hot with melted butter and warm honey or pure maple syrup. Makes 6-7 double waffles.

If there is waffle batter left over, store in refrigerator tightly covered. When ready to use, add a little milk and cook for thin pancakes or crepes.

Homemade Vanilla

3 vanilla beans
1 cup water, hot
2 Tbsp. honey
3 tsp. lecithin
3 tsp. safflower oil

Chop vanilla beans into small pieces. Combine beans with water in blender and mix. Pour into a small saucepan and bring to a boil. Remove from heat and store in a clean container with a tight lid. Leave overnight, then strain back into blender. Mix honey, lecithin, and oil and pour slowly into blender at a low speed. Pour into small containers and store in refrigerator.

Carrot Cake
(Sugarless, wheat-free)

5 egg yolks
1½ cups vegetable oil
1 cup honey
1 cup oat flour
1 cup rice flour
2 tsp. baking powder
1 tsp. cinnamon
1 tsp. coriander
1 tsp. salt
3 cups finely grated
   carrots (we use a
   nutmeg grater)

½ cup crushed pecans
   (optional)
5 egg whites
Frosting:
2 cups whipping cream
3 Tbsp. honey
2 tsp. vanilla
1 cup pecans (Reserve 12
   whole pecans for
   decorating top of cake.)

Beat egg yolks, add oil and honey, mixing well. Sift all dry
ingredients together and mix into liquids a little at a time.
Stir in grated carrots.

Beat egg whites until stiff and fold gently into batter.
Pour into three 9″ cake pans—grease and flour the bottoms
only. Cake will rise more easily if it doesn't have to climb a
greased wall. Bake in 300° oven for 50-60 minutes. Remove
from oven and cool. Put the three layers together with the
sweetened whipped cream and swirl over top and sides.

Crush and roll pecans in a plastic bag with a rolling pin.
Cover sides of cake with the rolled nuts. Evenly distribute
the 12 whole pecans on top. Refrigerate until serving time.
Serves 12.

Fresh Orange Marmalade

3 oranges   1 tsp. vanilla
1 cup honey

Scrub oranges with a stiff brush under running water. With a rind peeler, remove several strips of rind from each orange and place in a saucepan. Cut off remaining rind and discard. Dice oranges into small pieces, reserving all the juice. Add to pan and pour in honey and vanilla. Warm thoroughly over low heat and keep warm until serving. Serve in small pitcher that has been scalded and is hot. This is delicious served with waffles, pancakes, and muffins. Cool and use as topping for cottage cheese, yogurt, or homemade ice cream.

Variations: Add ¼ cup unsweetened fresh or canned pineapple or 1 ripe peach, chopped.

CHAPTER NINE

The 'Claws' That Refresh

The life of the flesh is in the blood.—Leviticus 17:11

At 48, the school administrator thought he had the world by the tail. He was tall, strong, only five pounds over his ideal weight, and he kept himself fit with clean habits.

"You have an excellent heart," his doctor told him one night. "If I were you, I'd take your wife out to dinner and celebrate."

"Matter of fact," Jim replied, "that's exactly what we're going to do."

The evening came and went pleasantly for the happy midwestern couple, but the night was a different story. Approximately twelve hours after his doctor told him he was in perfect health, a massive coronary attack stabbed Jim awake and left him gasping for breath.

In the ambulance the attendant turned to Mrs. Webster and said, "Your husband is dying. Are you certain you want to make the long trip to Memorial?"

"No," she said, "take him to the nearest hospital. Perhaps it will make the difference."

The speedy treatment saved the husband and father of three boys from death in a sudden medical emergency. But the best prognosis was that he would live only about three months, and if he made it beyond that, he would only be able to handle menial desk work without the slightest exertion.

Special tests at a large cardiac institution produced the same dismal observation: "Forty percent of the heart's left ventricle has been damaged. Your husband has two blocked arteries. There is no way he can survive."

Other doctors and further tests showed the same severely scarred tissue, the same 30 percent mortality prediction, the same suggestion that bypass surgery might be elected if he would last three months and grow strong enough.

"What can I do for my husband?" Mrs. Webster asked.

"Nothing much, except to keep him resting comfortably," a doctor replied. "If you like, you can bring him in one day ahead of surgery and we can build him up."

Mrs. Webster looked at her husband. He was ghostly pale. The physician's promise to "build him up in one day" sounded preposterous, but she said nothing.

She began looking around for alternatives to surgery. Through the casual comment of another doctor she learned of a process called "chelation" (kē-lā-shun), a relatively new treatment for heart patients. It successfully reduces deposits of calcium in the arteries and in other parts of the body. The term comes from the Greek word *chele* which refers to the claws of a lobster or crab. The amino acid used in chelation—disodium ethylenediamine tetraacetic acid (EDTA)—is inserted drop by drop into the bloodstream. Like pincers, the acid grabs the offending chemical substances and binds them to a bivalent metal or other mineral. "The therapy incorporates a metal or a mineral ion into a heterocyclic ring structure," says Bruce Halstead, M.D., of Health and Medical Group, Loma Linda, California.

The chemicals in chelation take hold of calcium with this clawlike manipulation. They encircle these minerals by a sophisticated reaction, destroying the toxic properties of the dangerous deposits. When the chemicals from chelation come in contact with the calcium or heavy metal, the enemy substances are bound, then excreted from the body through the kidneys.

Since no known cases of death or illness have been reported from chelation patients, Mrs. Webster decided to order it for Jim. For a long month they endured the time-consuming preliminary tests and twenty bottles of EDTA (treatments) for the first series. Finally color began to return to her husband's face. More treatments followed. "Your husband is going to be well," the doctor told Mrs. Webster. She guarded her emotions carefully, allowing herself only a glimmer of hope.

In three months Jim was up and moving about. Seven months after his heart attack, and after taking three series in the chelation therapy, he was talking about returning to work. Just to be certain of his recovery, Mrs. Webster arranged for exhaustive tests at a cardiac specialty center and decided not to tell the doctor about Jim's experience with chelation.

"I'm sorry," the doctor in charge told her, "I can't touch your husband until you fill me in on the details of his background."

"If you promise not to be prejudiced . . ."

"Well, I won't sign any work slips until I'm satisfied that he's in good health," the doctor assured her.

"Agreed," said Mrs. Webster. "That's exactly why I brought Jim here."

The entire test, including the treadmill examination, gave the doctor what he needed to pronounce the cardiac patient completely ready to return to work.

"When?" asked Mrs. Webster.

"Tomorrow, if he wishes," the doctor said.

Doctors at the first cardiac research institution who had examined Jim following his heart attack were baffled and amazed by the recovery of their patient. Today Jim is riding a bicycle, hiking, playing tennis—doing all the things he enjoys in leisure hours from work. He is on a maintenance schedule of chelation therapy and follows a good diet low in saturated fats, high in protein, and without sugar. "If the meat flies or swims we eat it," Mrs. Webster told us. "But we eat nothing prepared by man. Occasionally we eat rabbit if it's fresh."

A pastor swallows the sword

For thirty years the Reverend Daniel Cleveland built his evangelistic center into a thriving fellowship of 600 members. His hunting and fishing trips grew less and less frequent as he poured his heart and soul into the work of the church.

In 1968 at the age of sixty-six Pastor Cleveland was struck down by a massive coronary attack. The illness kept him on his back for six weeks and out of the pulpit for half a year. In 1969 he suffered a second heart attack which took him again to within a flicker of death.

"I learned about chelation shortly after that second attack," he told us. "Since then I've taken a total of forty treatments. After twenty treatments my blood pressure returned to normal (120/72) and my pulse stabilized at 80 with no skips." Ten more chelation treatments during the next year and ten more on the eve of his seventy-fourth birthday left him feeling as fit as he had ever felt.

"A while back I was big game hunting in Colorado," he recalled during our interview. "I went up to 13,000 feet without any problem. Next month I'm going to Arkansas to hunt and fish."

Pastor Cleveland knows of people coming from as far away as Mexico for the rejuvenating treatments that chemically clean out tired arteries filled with calcium and other deposits, making the body feel young again.

Nature's own chelation

All chelation isn't done with the arm on a pillow receiving liquid through a needle from a bottle overhead. Chelation is actually the important natural function occurring within living organisms of plants and animals all the time. Through chelation, plants and animals are able to use inorganic minerals. Chlorophyll, the green substance in plants, is a chelate of magnesium. Hemoglobin, the red blood cell pigment which carries oxygen in the blood, is a chelate of iron. Chelation plays an important role in the formation and function of enzymes, the protein which controls most of the body's vital functions.

"Most of the successful drugs which are used in the treatment of disease are dependent upon the chelation process for their action," says Dr. Bruce W. Halstead, who supplied the basic information for this report. "Chelation processes comprise some of the most complex chemical reactions found in nature, and are the mechanisms which control many body functions. These same principles are used in chelation therapy to treat arteriosclerosis and related diseases.[1]

These dramatic testimonials by reputable medical clinics may tend to label the therapy a cure-all, but of course such is not the case. It simply removes abnormal deposits of calcium from which other diseases originate.

Routing enemy number one

Hardening of the arteries (arteriosclerosis) is Western man's most serious enemy. In 1974 alone it took the lives of approximately one million people.

Several different types of the disease are on record, the most common being atherosclerosis (fatty substances deposited in and beneath the inner artery wall). This closes off the flow of blood, thus starving the whole body. When this happens all kinds of serious problems arise, including stroke, high blood pressure, diabetes, kidney disorders, senility, thyroid and adrenal disturbances, emphysema, and Parkinson's disease. When an organ is robbed of its blood supply the bodily part can't get required nutrients and oxygen, and toxic wastes cannot be removed. Eventually the organ becomes diseased and the person dies.

We usually associate arteriosclerosis with the aging process, but it actually begins in early childhood. Not until the diameter of the blood vessel is reduced by more than 50 percent are the effects noticed. Sometimes the artery can be 70 percent closed without drastic results.

Another form of arteriosclerosis occurs when calcium is deposited within the media of the larger arteries. Chelation is effective in eliminating the dangerous mineral components of the diseased arteries which have adversely affected the enzyme systems of the arterial lining.

The risk that exists

No type of medical procedure is without a degree of risk. Chelation is no exception. Hundreds of thousands of treatments have been administered without unpleasant reactions, but each person seeking information about the process should know of the potential hazards involved.

The EDTA is administered intravenously, making it nontoxic. This generally produces no serious side effects.

Occasionally thrombophlebitis has resulted. Occasionally too there is pain where the injection is made, but this can be rapidly controlled. If the infusion is done too rapidly the muscle may cramp. The kidneys may be irritated because of the heavy excretory load as the undesirable chemicals are flushed out of the body. Transient fever, joint aches, headaches, loss of appetite, nausea, fatigue, and extreme thirst are occasional symptoms to be endured. Allergic reactions have been known to occur, along with sneezing, nasal congestion, dizziness, and skin rash. But these are nothing when compared with the danger of leaving the deadly chemicals in the body to keep the blood from doing its work.

EDTA and the AMA

The American Medical Association does not endorse chelation therapy completely because it has ruled its effects as "not lasting." The AMA is officially on record as considering the uses of EDTA as being "investigational."

One reason that the treatment is temporary is that the patient often holds on to poor eating habits. Like machinery, human beings need periodic checkups and repairs. The U.S. Food and Drug Administration has approved EDTA for use in chelating heavy metals and digitalis intoxication. The AMA's charge that chelation is "investigative" doesn't imply that human beings are being used as guinea pigs. The records in favor of chelation accumulating in the files of the American Academy of Medical Preventics (the medical specialty group establishing standards and a continuing evaluation of chelation therapy) are piling up in impressive numbers.

Preparation for chelation

Before the treatment, the patient undergoes a thorough medical and laboratory workup. If the tests show that the patient should have the treatment, the procedure begins on an outpatient basis.

One treatment is administered, followed by a three-day rest. If no bad reactions are noticed, the patient starts his full course of twenty treatments requiring three to four hours each. A qualified physician must supervise the treatments. In rare cases, fifty treatments are required, but the usual number is twenty.

Other forms of treatment

There are other forms of treatment for arteriosclerosis. Surgery is one. A surgical excision or stripping of the atheromatous intimal lining of some of the larger arteries is common. Bypass surgery can often create a new vascular blood supply to circumvent a blocked coronary artery. In generalized atherosclerotic condition, surgery is usually ineffective.

Chelation therapy is usually safer than surgery. It's also less expensive and promotes the health of the entire circulatory system. Surgery is limited to only one segment of the arterial system.

Many are the testimonies of the value of this relatively new method of rejuvenating the engine of your priceless machine.

THINGS TO DO

1. Regardless of the success of chelation, always remember: prevention is far better than treatment.

2. Use only polyunsaturated oils in your diet. Avoid rich desserts. Take lecithin daily.

3. Be persistent in efforts to find help through chelation if local medical counselors fail to help.

4. Arrange for regular exercise to keep your heart and arteries healthy.

5. Use food wisely, beginning with the recipes at the end of this chapter.

Lecithin can save your life

This natural, vital food, made from defatted soybeans, is one of the latest discoveries in the quest for elements to help prolong life.

Lecithin breaks down or dissolves hard fat cells or cholesterol. Some doctors call it the heart saver because it prevents hardening of the arteries (atherosclerosis) caused by a buildup of cholesterol in the blood.

It's found in all body cells—particularly in the brain and nerve cells. Taking it as a supplement is particularly beneficial in diets for diabetes, heart disease, multiple sclerosis, nephritis, psoriasis, lowering high blood pressure, and reducing as well as preventing gall stones.

Physicians use lecithin to help keep blood from clotting in the arteries. Lecithin also creates a greater resistance to virus infection. Evidence shows that lecithin can immunize against pneumonia.

Some medical research reports advise taking liquid lecithin, which requires lesser amounts than the other forms. It looks like honey, but is tasteless. Take with a tart juice drink to prevent its sticking to the roof of the mouth.

Generally, lecithin helps the body to enjoy vibrant good health and provides surges of strength that make the day's work lighter. Lecithin is found in liver, whole grains, soybeans, raw nuts, sunflower seeds, and squash seeds. Eggs are also an excellent source of lecithin.

Mentally and physically, you'll be better off with adequate supplies of lecithin in your diet. Many doctors prescribe two to four tablespoons of soy lecithin daily.

Unsaturating the Butter

Blend 1 lb. butter with 1 cup safflower oil (or other polyunsaturated oil).

Add 2 Tbsp. soy lecithin granules or liquid.

Blend together well and place in a plastic container with a tight lid.

This will give you the taste and spreading quality of butter with fewer chemicals than margarine and less saturated fat than butter.

"Pure" oil does not mean the same thing to the manufacturer and the government as it does to you. The Federal Drug Administration allows the manufacturer to print "pure oil" on the label if he began with pure oil, even though he has added a variety of chemicals and foreign matter.

Sunshine Tea

Fill glass gallon jug with cold water. Add 4 tea bags. Set in warm sunshine and leave all day. Chill and serve over ice. Garnish with lemon wedges and fresh mint leaves. This can also be used for hot tea. Tea made in this manner will not be bitter.

The Queen's Tea

½ cup pearl barley   2 lemons
2½ quarts hot water   6 oranges

Rinse barley in cold water and drain. Cover with hot water and bring to a simmer. Allow to simmer 1 hour. Strain. While still hot add the rind of one lemon and the rind of three oranges. Cool at room temperature and strain. Add the juice of the lemons and the oranges. Chill.

According to one of the cooks in the royal family of England, the Queen Mother, Queen Elizabeth, and Princess Margaret drink this beverage often. They are known for their beautiful complexions and some say it is due in part to this drink.

Red Wine Vinegar Dressing

½ tsp. salt   ¼ tsp. paprika
¼ tsp. black pepper   ⅓ cup red wine vinegar
¼ tsp. dry mustard   ¾ cup safflower oil or corn
¼ tsp. sweet basil   oil
¼ tsp. oregano

Mix seasonings together in a small dish. Crush basil and oregano hard with the back of a spoon to release the flavors and refine the leaves. (Mortar and pestle would work great here.) Pour vinegar into a jar or cruet and add the seasonings. Cover jar tightly and shake vigorously until blended. Add oil to vinegar mixture and shake again, mixing well. Chill and allow flavors to blend in refrigerator. At serving time shake again. This amount can be blended into a commercial-size cruet that is available in supermarkets. No cholesterol. No sugar. If your sweet tooth hasn't adjusted yet to tart dressings, add a dash of artificial sweetener.

Homemade Catsup

¼ cup cider vinegar
¼ cup tarragon vinegar
¼ cup pure honey
3 cups tomatoes
2 cups tomato paste
¼ tsp. cloves
¼ tsp. onion salt
¼ tsp. garlic salt
¼ tsp. celery salt
2 tsp. cinnamon
1 tsp. allspice
1 Tbsp. salt

Combine all the ingredients in a saucepan and simmer over low heat for 10 minutes. Cool. Pour into glass containers that have gone through a dishwasher sanitary cycle or jars that have been boiled for 10 minutes and cooled. Refrigerate immediately.

Supermarket varieties of catsup are made with sugar and chemicals to give them longer shelf life. Diabetics and hypoglycemics will especially appreciate this recipe. However, everyone would be better off with less sugar and preservatives in their diet.

Chiang Chicken Salad

5 cups cooked diced
  chicken
½ cup crushed soy nuts
1 cup sliced water
  chestnuts
½ cup diagonally sliced
  celery
½ cup diagonally sliced
  green onions
1½—2 cups fresh cut
  pineapple (or
  unsweetened canned)
1 large can chow mein
  noodles
Dressing:
1 cup sour cream
1 cup mayonnaise
1 Tbsp. soy sauce
1 tsp. curry powder
3 Tbsp. chutney
1 scant tsp. salt

Toss together the chicken, nuts, vegetables and fruit. Pour dressing over the salad and mix well. Chill until serving. Now add the noodles and toss again. Serves 8-10.

Zesty Zucchini Casserole

1 cup brown rice
2⅔ cups water
1 tsp. salt
1 Tbsp. oil
4 med. zucchini
3 med. tomatoes, sliced
1 lb. grated Jack cheese
2 cups sour cream

1 4-oz. can Ortega green
 chiles, chopped
1 Tbsp. parsley
2 Tbsp. green pepper
2 Tbsp. green onion
1 tsp. oregano
1 tsp. garlic salt
½ tsp. pepper

Bring water to a boil with salt. Add rice and oil. Cook over low heat until rice is tender, 45-50 minutes. When done, spread rice in a 13″ × 9″ pyrex baking dish. Cover with the thinly sliced zucchini, a layer of grated cheese (½ the amount), and a layer of the sliced tomatoes. Mix sour cream, vegetables, and seasonings together. Pour over tomatoes and top with the remaining grated cheese. Bake for 30 minutes in a moderate 350° oven.

Delicious served with a fruit salad.

Korean Salad

1 lb. fresh spinach, rinsed
 well
1 lb. fresh bean sprouts
1 5-oz. can water chestnuts
2 hard cooked eggs,
 chopped

Dressing:
1 cup soy oil (or vegetable
 oil)
¼ cup wine vinegar
⅓ cup catsup or tomato
 sauce
2 Tbsp. honey or other
 sweetener

Break spinach into bite-size pieces in your salad bowl. Add bean sprouts and chestnuts. Mix dressing ingredients together well and pour over salad. Toss. Sprinkle with chopped eggs. Serve immediately.

Mushroom Stroganoff

2 Tbsp. butter
1 medium onion, finely chopped
1 clove garlic, grated fine
3 Tbsp. fresh parsley, minced
2-3 cups fresh mushrooms, halved or quartered, depending on size

1 cup cottage cheese
½ cup powdered milk
½ cup plain yogurt
1 egg, slightly beaten

In saucepan melt butter and add the onion and garlic. Sauté until clear but not brown. Add parsley and mushrooms and cook over low heat about five minutes, stirring often. Mix cheese, milk, yogurt, and egg together. Add to vegetables and keep on heat just long enough to heat through. Sprinkle with salt and pepper. Serve hot over steaming brown rice or hot buttered spinach noodles.

Quesadillas

½ lb. Jack cheese, grated
½ lb. Longhorn cheese, grated
¼ cup finely diced onion

1 dozen flour tortillas
1 ripe avocado
2 medium tomatoes
alfalfa sprouts

Toss the cheeses and onion together. Place 6 tortillas out flat on baking sheet and spread generously with cheese. Place under broiler and cook until bubbly.

Serve with sliced avocados, sliced tomatoes, and alfalfa sprouts. This may be served flat and eaten with a knife and fork or folded over and eaten with the hands like a taco.

CHAPTER TEN

The Cleansing Fast

Instead of using medicine, fast a day.—Plutarch, c. A.D. 46-120

The subject of fasting might seem out of place in a book on nutrition, but careful abstention can offer physical, mental, and spiritual rewards to those who have the discipline to practice it.

Nutrition is the series of processes by which food is changed into living tissues. Fasting is a method of cleansing the body from toxins built up over a long period. During the fast, the body seems to gain new reserves of energy. Unhealthful weight is burned off, and the arteries are cleaned out.

The mental rewards are almost immediate. Just as a full stomach produces a sluggish brain, an empty stomach enlightens the mind. People who fast are more aware of their spiritual needs and more perceptive in all five senses of the body.

Spiritually, fasting denies the body so that the spirit may be strengthened. "Fasting," writes Arthur Wallis in his book *God's Chosen Fast* (Christian Literature Crusade), "has a way of detaching us from the world of material, so that our thinking becomes rightly orientated, focused on God, and the unseen world of which He is the center. This inevitably results in a release of faith...."[1]

Mr. Wallis sees three kinds of fasts in the Scriptures: (1) the normal fast (only water, no food); (2) the absolute fast (no water or food); and (3) the partial fast (observing certain dietary restrictions rather than complete abstention). (The absolute fast should not be undertaken, however. It is too dangerous.)

Many of the greatest personalities of history observed the fast. Among those who fasted were Moses, who gave the law; David, who reigned long and successfully as Israel's king; Elijah, whose accomplishments as a prophet were among the most astonishing; and Daniel, the seer.

The Lord Jesus Christ himself provided an example in fasting. After he was led into the wilderness he fasted forty days and forty nights. Only *afterward* was he hungry (Matthew 4:2). Jesus never commanded his followers to fast. He rather *assumed* that they would. He instructed his disciples, "...*when* you fast," not "...*if* you fast" (Matthew 6:16).

Throughout the history of the Church, fasting has been practiced by great Christian leaders. Among them are Reformers such as Luther, Calvin, and Knox. Fasting was never confined to a single school of theology, denomination, or nation. This scriptural teaching should not be overlooked by Christians today.

The self-fueling machine

Even some people with no theological basis for fasting have entered into the practice eagerly and with profit:

The novelist Upton Sinclair, who fasted often during his

ninety years, said: "I have found a perfect health, a new state of existence, a feeling of purity and happiness, something unknown to humans...."

Leo Tolstoy of Russia and his literary cronies fasted in order to rid their minds of materialistic concerns and to rest their stomachs.

In ancient Greece some fasted to sharpen their minds and to make their bodies pure.

Physicians testify that patients suffering from schizophrenia have found relief after fasting, followed by observance of new dietary habits.

Four hundred years before the birth of Christ, Hippocrates, the father of modern medicine, declared, "Everyone has a doctor in him. We just have to help him in his work." He added: "To eat when you are sick is to feed your sickness."

The ultimate diet

In a weight-conscious society most Americans (seventy-five million of whom are overweight) view fasting as a method of dieting to shed unsightly pounds. A book by Allan Cott, M.D., popularized   the phrase "the ultimate diet" to describe the fast for dieters.[2]

Before going on a fast to lose weight, you should consult your physician. Some people should never fast. Among them are children or adolescents, thin persons, mental patients, pregnant mothers and women who have just given birth, diabetics, heart patients, and hypoglycemics.

Whether you wish it or not, one result of fasting is the loss of weight. The palate becomes more sensitive to tastes, and skin problems will tend to heal. The eyes light up with extra alertness. The body looks and feels younger and the person likes himself for having the courage to get control of his appetites.

The credo of the famous Buchinger Clinics in Germany and Spain, published by Abbott Laboratories in Chicago, states:

> We must restore fasting to the place it occupied in an ancient hierarchy of values "above medicine." We must rediscover it and restore it to honor because it is a necessity. A beneficial fast of several weeks, as practiced in the earliest days of the Church, was to give strength, life, and health to the body and soul of all Christians who had the courage to practice it.

Saving on food means saving on money when you fast. You also save time which can be spent in other pursuits. Coffee habits are broken during a fast; the shackles of smoking and drinking of alcoholic beverages, and drug dependency can be snapped; sleep is deeper and more restful; tensions lessen; blood pressure falls, as do cholesterol levels.

Fasting moves the lever of spiritual power as well. Author Wallis advocates the technique of the fast to stay well through proper nutrition.

"A new day is dawning," he states, "and a new thirst for the Spirit is beginning to awaken the slumbering Church."

Water or juice?

There are at least two approaches to fasting—one with water only, the other with juice only. Paavo O. Airola, author of *How to Keep Slim, Healthy and Young with Juice Fasting* believes strongly in the juice fast. He states:

> Although the old, classic form of fasting was a pure water fast, all the leading fasting authorities today agree that juice fasting is far superior to a water fast.

Perhaps, if the effective way of making raw vegetable
and fruit juices were known before, the healers of the
past would have used them, too. I have supervised
both types of fasting and I agree with Dr. Otto
Buchinger, Jr., who has supervised more fasts than
any other doctor, that fasting on fresh raw juices of
fruits and vegetables, plus vegetable broths and herb
teas, results in much faster recovery from disease and
more effective cleansing and rejuvenation of the tissues than does the traditional water fast. There are
hundreds of clinics in Germany alone where fasting is
a number one method of healing. And all of them use
juice fasting exclusively.[3]

Many persons have developed the healthful habit of fasting one day a week. This is a practice we heartily endorse
and practice. If you choose to fast for only one day a week
the water fast is quite acceptable. And breaking the fast is
simply eating as usual, in more moderation. Longer fasts,
however, seem to require the safety margin of juice.

A world-renowned authority on nutrition and biochemistry, Dr. Ragnar Berg, says about the superiority of juice
fasting over water fasting:

During fasting the body burns up and excretes huge
amounts of accumulated wastes. We can help this
cleansing process by drinking alkaline juices instead
of water while fasting. I have supervised many fasts
and made extensive examinations and tests of fasting
patients, and I am convinced that drinking alkali-
forming fruit and vegetable juices, instead of water,
during fasting will increase the healing effect of fasting. Elimination of uric acid and other inorganic acids
will be accelerated. And sugars in juices will
strengthen the heart.... Juice fasting is, therefore, the
best form of fasting.

You should consult an expert before you fast longer than a week. Then after a few weeks on a diet with priority foods you may try fasting again. Do not begin a fasting period without studying what you are doing and don't begin without spiritual preparation.

The physical benefits of fasting are perhaps more obvious, but the spiritual accomplishments may be even greater. God may guide you to portions of Scripture that are appropriate for this particular experience and bring about dramatic and dynamic changes in you and in those for whom you pray.

Because it was recommended by a fasting supervisor, we have found that the following cleansing diet is the best preparation for fasting beyond twenty-four hours:

1. Two days of two meals only.
2. The first meal in midmorning consisting of an abundance of raw fruits in season; the afternoon or evening meal of raw vegetables in season, with oil and vinegar if desired.

On the day you begin

Consume a minimum of two quarts (64 oz.) of liquids the first day and the following days. The variety listed below is suggested for the juice fast, to be taken periodically throughout the day between mild exercise, rest, and normal activity. The activity must not be of the highly stressful type:

2 cups of herb tea (8 oz. each)	16 oz.
1 cup fresh vegetable juice	8 oz.
1 cup vegetable broth or vegetable juice	8 oz.
1 cup fresh juice diluted 50/50 with water, taken on arising	8 oz.
1 cup freshly squeezed fruit juice	8 oz.
1 cup vegetable broth at bedtime	8 oz.
	56 oz.

The remaining 8 oz. needed are to be consumed by drinking mineral water, if available. When thirsty, drink more water.

Breaking the long fast

Use moderation ... moderation ... moderation.
• Only small amounts of food should be eaten on the first three days after fasting.
• Food should be eaten slowly and chewed for a long time.
• Drink the same fasting liquids on the first day, but add a raw fruit in the morning and fresh vegetable soup at night.
• On the second day, drink the liquids of the fast but add prunes for breakfast, fresh green salad for lunch, and vegetable soup at night. Eat two pieces of fresh fruit between meals.
• The third day should be similar to the second, but adding yogurt or kefir in the morning. Have larger salad at noon with a vegetable. Add a serving of cottage cheese, whole-grain bread and butter with the vegetable soup in the evening.
• On the fourth day resume normal eating but don't return to the eating of nonessential foods.
Paavo Airola, in his controversial book *How to Get Well* (Health Plus, Phoenix) offers the following tips on making the most from your fasting:
1. Enemas are an absolute must. They will assist the body in its cleansing and detoxifying effort by washing out all the toxic wastes from the system.
2. Drugs should be eliminated except those used for heart disease, diabetes, and arthritis. Of course this will have been checked with your doctor.

3. Vitamins should be discontinued except in special cases.

4. No smoking or drinking. Many have experienced total healing from these disease-causing habits after two weeks of fasting.

5. Juices should be made fresh just before drinking.

6. Herb teas especially recommended are: peppermint, rose hips, and camomile.

7. Work should go on as usual unless it is heavy construction-type work.

8. Exercise should include walking in the fresh air to assist in cleansing of the blood and tissues.

9. A daily bath is imperative as one third of all body impurities and wastes are eliminated through the skin.

10. Positive attitude is essential. Have confidence in what you are doing.

Avoid black coffee and tea during your fast. These only stimulate your central nervous system when you are trying to give them a rest. Anything such as a diet drink that recalls the sensation of eating or drinking food should be avoided.

Plan for periods of meditation and prayer. During your fast, arrange for at least an hour of exercise each day. This will reduce, rather than stimulate, your appetite. Hike, play golf, ride a bicycle, swim—do all the things you enjoy doing.

Dr. Cott tells of a Russian who was entering the twenty-fifth day of a fast when he met him. The Slav testified that he had never felt better, and that he was happy about the weight he had lost while he continued his full work load, drinking only water.

As toxins leave the body, new spurts of energy may reward the one who fasts. The mind is quickened and the senses all become sharp. An adage states: "A full stomach does not like to think." With the one who fasts, the opposite is true.

During your fast, avoid quick movements, like getting up suddenly or leaping out of bed. Your reduced blood pressure might result in dizziness.

The discipline of going without food should always be linked to a purpose—a spiritual exercise. When this is done, the first pangs of hunger will not be overwhelming.

Should you fast? No one can prescribe for another. It is a most individual decision. But when done with a purpose, even the practice of taking no food can help keep you well.

THINGS TO DO

1. See a doctor before a lengthy fast.

2. Fast with spiritual goals in view.

3. Consider the long fast as a therapeutic approach to maladies. Consult the experts. Don't do it without counsel and study.

4. Use the fast to help control weight.

5. Use the time and money you have gained through fasting to help the hungry in your community and elsewhere in the starving world.

Homemade Stock

Stock to some people means a can, a tablespoon, or a cube of bouillon. Others opt for a can of consommé. These represent instant taste in a can. But if you want a genuine, fresh stock, like that served in an exceptionally fine restaurant, you can have it. And it's not difficult, although it will take a little time. The rewards are worth the effort.

Forget your past recipes that have started out with bones and water. There is only one way to make superb stock. You must begin with bones and roasting.

Brown stock method

Buy from your butcher 5 lbs. of beef or veal bones. Have him crack them. If the bones are lean, ask for a little fat.

First rinse the bones in a pan of salty water. Salt is a cleanser and this rinse will give the bones a fresh smell. Pat dry with a paper towel. Place the bones and fat in a large baking pan and roast them for 2 hours in a hot 425° oven. Occasionally turn them and enjoy the marvelous aroma. Halfway through, add a couple of large onions and half a dozen carrots. Roast until everything is brown but not too dark. The vegetables will give the stock a rich color. Put your tea kettle on and have boiling water available for the next step. Place the bones in a large kettle and pour the boiling water into the roasting pan. Scrape every drop of flavoring off the surface. Pour into the kettle and rinse the pan again if necessary. Use enough water to cover the bones.

Add 2 Tbsp. cider vinegar (this helps release nutrients from the bones), two bay leaves, a stalk of celery cut into several pieces, a dash of sweet basil, a dash of salt, and a few peppercorns. Cover tightly and simmer over low heat for 3½ to 4 hours. If the taste is not rich enough, simmer a little longer with the lid off. This is not soup for the table but a rich stock that will enhance many dishes for you.

Stir well. Pour through a strainer into the containers for storage. We use a 1½-pint plastic freezer container (3 cups) and freeze immediately. Save some for refrigerator storage and use within a week. The fat will rise during cooling and storage—this gives a layer of protection to the broth. Skim off before using.

Poultry or white stock method

Accumulate bones from cooked turkey or chicken. Example: If you have baked chicken breasts and boned them for using the meat in a salad or a casserole, save the bones. If you don't have enough to cover a roasting pan, put them in the freezer and keep until you prepare chicken again. With a good-sized turkey you will have enough bones to roast. If the bones are taken from your family's plates, rinse the bones with boiling water, pat dry with a paper towel, and freeze or roast.

Roast your collection of bones with 2 large onions and 6 fresh carrots in a large pan in a hot 425° oven for 1 hour. (If you begin with raw bones, perhaps after boning chicken breasts for baking, you can bake for a longer period.) Turn at least twice during roasting. When all are nicely browned, place in kettle. Pour boiling water into the roasting pan and scrape all the drippings off and add to kettle. Stir in 2 Tbsp. cider vinegar, 2 bay leaves, 1 stalk celery cut up, a dash of sweet basil, a dash of salt, and a few peppercorns. Cover and simmer over low heat for 3½ to 4 hours. Follow directions as above.

Now you have stock that will give you superb soups, gravies, or sauces.

You don't have to use 5 lbs. of bones. One pound of bones and scrap meat and 4 cups of water and seasonings will provide one or two cups of beautiful broth. That's a nice amount to freeze if you're not ready to use it.

It is imperative to have a gelatinous stock if you want a superior soup. If you can slice your soup when it is cold you have achieved the ultimate and have mastered the soup pot. Now use that sensational stock for nourishing soups for your family. Use the poultry stock for poultry soups, vegetable soups, and pepper pot. Use the brown stock for minestrone and other hearty soups. Use it also in small amounts for stroganoff.

Have it handy for adding to the drippings of a roasted turkey. First pour in enough hot water to release the tasty morsels and scrape pan well. Then add your stock to expand the quantity. Simmer and reduce quantity for a rich, full flavor. When you have a beef roast do the same, but use your brown stock. You may want to use 2 pints, reducing the amount in an open pan as the stock browns. This will be gravy fit for a king.

Remember, use stock, not water. Any liquid added to a recipe should be tasty on its own.

Chilled Beet Soup

1 lb. small fresh beets, w/skin
1 cup water
1 tsp. onion salt

1 quart fresh and well-chilled buttermilk
1 Tbsp. dill weed

Cook beets in 1 cup water over low heat until tender. Peel and place in blender. Add any remaining liquid from pan and whiz until smooth. Add salt. Blend in the buttermilk and dill weed. Serve in cold bowls for six or eight. Garnish with a watercress sprig.

Fresh Pea Soup

2 cups boiling water
1 cup cashew nuts (for thickener)
½ tsp. garlic salt
½ tsp. onion salt

1 Tbsp. corn oil
3 cups poultry stock
1 lb. fresh or frozen shelled peas
dash of crushed oregano

Pour water into blender and add nuts, salt, and oil. Blend until smooth. Add poultry stock and fresh peas. Whiz until mixture is again smooth. Pour into saucepan and heat until hot. Sprinkle in a dash of crushed oregano and stir. Serve immediately.

Vera Deyneka's Russian Borscht

4 qts. meat broth*
  (chicken, beef, or pork)
1 bay leaf
3 potatoes, chopped
5 carrots, chopped
Season with salt, if needed
½ stick butter
1 small head cabbage,
  shredded

1 medium white onion,
  chopped
1 Tbsp. fresh parsley,
  minced
1 Tbsp. dill weed, fresh or
  dried
1 bunch large beets (3-5)
1 Tbsp. honey
1 Tbsp. lemon juice

Place prepared broth in large kettle and add bay leaf, potatoes, carrots, and seasoning. Simmer for one hour. Melt butter and add cabbage, onion, parsley, and dill weed. Fry lightly and add to soup. Simmer for another hour. Cook beets in minimum amount of water over low heat until tender. Cool slightly, peel and grate into soup. Add honey and lemon. Simmer another 30 minutes. Serve hot with a dollop of sour cream on top of each serving.

*(This broth is made the day before so all fat can be skimmed off. See page 210 for directions.) This soup is the special preparation of Vera Demidovich Deyneka, a peasant girl from Cherniyevichi, who became the wife of world-renowned Peter Deyneka, a Russian evangelist. Mrs. Deyneka has made hundreds of gallons of this traditional Slavic food.

Vegetable Tonic

1 cup tomato juice
1 cup cabbage juice
1 cup sprouted alfalfa seed

2 cups fresh celery juice
dash of salt
squeeze of lemon

Make juices separately in blender. Then mix together and serve immediately. You do not need to strain this.

California Cantaloupe Drink

1 medium cantaloupe,
peeled and chilled
2 cups milk
2 eggs

2 Tbsp. malt powder
2 Tbsp. powdered milk
1 Tbsp. lemon juice

Put cantaloupe pulp, seeds and the netlike fiber attached to the seeds in the blender. Whiz at high speed, strain, and set aside. In blender mix milk, eggs, powders, and lemon juice. Pour in pureed cantaloupe. Serve immediately. Makes two large or four small servings.

Emerald Rain

1 ripe banana
2 cups pineapple juice
1 cup ice water

½ cup alfalfa sprouts
¼ cup watercress

Place all ingredients into the blender and liquefy for 2 minutes. Drink immediately or chill and use the same day.

Joanne's Broccoli Salad

1 lb. fresh broccoli
½ lb. fresh mushrooms
one medium red onion
Dressing: vinegar & oil
1 large clove garlic

1 cup safflower or olive oil
½ cup wine vinegar
1 tsp. salt
1 Tbsp. sesame seed

Select the freshest broccoli you can find. Wash well and trim off the heavy stalks. Break broccoli into flowerets and place in container that can be covered—preferably stainless steel or plastic. Rinse mushrooms quickly, trim and slice into broccoli. Peel onion and cut in half. Slice in very thin strips and toss with other vegetables.

Crush garlic through a garlic press or grate until fine. Mix with the oil and vinegar in a jar and shake vigorously. Add salt and sesame seeds.

A to Z Salad

1 avocado, choose in advance so it can ripen
1 head cauliflower, broken into flowerets
1 red onion, sliced thin
1 sprig fresh parsley
1 green bell pepper, thinly sliced
6 crisp zucchini, thinly sliced

Set avocado aside for garnish. Combine all the vegetables in a stainless steel bowl or a salad bowl. Pour warm dressing over vegetables and place in the refrigerator several hours before serving. Toss well and garnish bowl with slices of avocado.

Dressing:
1 cup vegetable oil
1 cup wine vinegar
1 Tbsp. salt
1 tsp. celery seed
1 tsp. dry mustard
1 tsp. paprika

Mix all ingredients together in a saucepan and bring to a boil. Cool slightly.

Cindy's Spinach Salad

½ to ¾ lb. spinach, rinsed well
½ head iceberg lettuce
4 hard-cooked eggs, each cut into four wedges
1 cup croutons
¼ lb. Swiss cheese, shredded
¼ lb. Swiss cheese, cut into ¼" strips
2 ripe avocados, peeled and sliced
½ red onion, peeled and thinly sliced

In large salad bowl, break spinach and lettuce into bite-size pieces. Toss together. Add eggs, croutons, all the cheese, avocados, and red onion rings. Pour dressing over all ingredients and toss again. You may wish to pass the dressing and let each choose the amount desired.

Chinese Peas (Snow Peas)

1 Tbsp. soy oil
1 Tbsp. butter
½ tsp. salt
¼ tsp. white pepper
¼ tsp. sweet basil
1 lb. Chinese peas
1 stalk celery

Heat oil and butter with the seasonings. Rinse and carefully string the fresh peas. Cut celery diagonally into narrow strips. Add the vegetables to the oil mixture and cook over medium heat, stirring almost constantly for 5 minutes. They should remain crisp and be served immediately. If you wish, they can be added to cooked brown rice or buttered noodles.

Variation: Add bean sprouts and fresh sliced mushrooms. Eliminate the sweet basil and add 1 Tbsp. soy sauce.

Crab Bisque

1 can condensed tomato soup
1 can condensed celery soup
1 cup half and half
¼ tsp. thyme
1 7-8 oz. can crabmeat or pkg. frozen crabmeat
1 Tbsp. butter
dash of salt & pepper
¼ cup sherry
chopped chives

Whip the tomato soup and pour into saucepan. Whip the celery soup with the cream and add to the tomato soup with the thyme. Stir in the crabmeat, butter, salt, and pepper. Simmer 20 minutes. Add the sherry and simmer 10 more minutes. Serve hot, garnished with chives. Makes 4-6 servings.

One-Thousand-Calorie Diet

This is a doctor-recommended balanced diet which will cause a weight loss in most people. You do not need some exotic combination of foods to lose weight. You need determination. Good success to you!

BREAKFAST

Fruit	1 serving
Egg	1
Toast	1 whole-wheat slice
Skim milk	½ cup
Decaffeinated coffee or tea	no cream or sugar

LUNCH OR SUPPER

Cottage cheese	½ cup or 1 meat exchange
Vegetable—group I	½ cup
Vegetable—group I or II	½ cup
Bread	1 whole-wheat slice
Fruit	1 serving
Skim milk	1 cup
Decaffeinated coffee or tea	no cream or sugar

DINNER

Meat—lean	3 ounces or 3 meat exchanges
Vegetable—group I	½ cup
Vegetable—group II	½ cup
Bread	1 whole-wheat slice
Margarine	1 teaspoon
Fruit	1 serving
Skim milk	1 cup
Decaffeinated coffee or tea	no cream or sugar

FOODS ALLOWED

FRUITS (1 serving)

Apple	½ average
Applesauce	⅓ cup
Banana	½ small
Cantaloupe	½ average
Cherries	13 or 14
Grapefruit	½ large
Grapefruit juice	½ cup
Grapes	½ cup
Orange Juice	⅓ cup
Oranges	1 small
Other berries	½ cup
Peaches	1 small
Pear	1 small
Pineapple	⅓ cup
Plums	2 medium
Prunes	2 medium
Strawberries	¾ cup
Watermelon	½ cup diced

VEGETABLES

(½ cup) Group I

Asparagus	Lettuce
Broccoli	Radishes
Cabbage	Sauerkraut
Cauliflower	Spinach
Celery	Squash, summer
Cucumbers	
Greens (all kinds)	Tomatoes
	Tomato juice

(½ cup) Group II

Beans, green	Onions
Beans, wax	Peppers, green
Beets	
Brussel sprouts	Pumpkin
Carrots	Rutabagas
Okra	Squash, winter
	Turnips

MEAT (1 exchange)

Cottage cheese	½ cup
Egg	1
Roast chicken	1 slice
Meat	1 ounce
Yellow cheese	1 ounce

CHAPTER ELEVEN

Toward a Speedier Recovery

I treated him, God cured him.—Ambroise Paré, c. 1510-1590

In the corridors of most hospitals across the land, the skill of surgeons is superb and the dedication of the nursing staff is marvelously devoted and efficient. But a series of spot checks by the Chairman of the American Medical Society's Council on Food and Nutrition has found that some of these same skilled servants of the sick are either ignorant of, or downright indifferent to, the basic nutritional needs of recuperating patients in their care.

The AMA official, Charles E. Butterworth, M.D., said in a March/April 1974 article for *Nutrition Today* that the lack of therapy through nutrition is a scandal of national scope which he branded "inexcusable" and "tragic."

"It is well known," Dr. Butterworth said, "that malnutrition interferes with wound healing and increases susceptibility to infection. It thus becomes imperative to ensure that preventable malnutrition does not contribute to the mortality, morbidity, and prolonged bed-occupancy rates of our hospital population. So it's time to swing open the door and have a look at this skeleton in the hospital closet."

The AMA official documents his findings with a number of case histories. One involves a white male patient eighty years old suffering gangrene of the left foot and toes. For some twelve months previously, diagnosis showed small multiple brain-stem infarctions caused by arteriosclerosis. Swallowing was difficult for the patient, and he had eaten sparingly for several months before his admission. A surgical procedure followed and recovery was uneventful.

Some five weeks later the patient elected to have a gastrostomy to facilitate feeding. Eight days after the incision was made in his stomach, sutures were taken out; hours later the wound came open, spilling the abdominal contents. Doctors used general anesthesia and resutured the incision. There was no evidence whatever that healing had taken place.

No vitamin supplement had been prescribed for the patient up to this time. Now the man was started on an injectable multiple vitamin preparation. But the prescription did not contain folic acid, "the *only* vitamin in which the patient was then proved deficient," according to Dr. Butterworth. The patient had been given only glucose and salt up until this time.

On the following day a nutritionist observed that the patient was pale and drawn, covered with black and blue marks indicating that capillaries had broken. He was suffering from protein and calorie malnutrition. Tube feedings of a solution containing adequate protein were begun. He was also given injections of all vitamins, including high doses of vitamin C. Two weeks later the patient was nearly a well man and was discharged to go home.

The physician was surprised, he said, that so few of his associates comprehended the role of vitamins in recuperative therapy. When the body doesn't have enough vitamin

C, zinc, and protein available, injuries and surgical cuts can't heal properly. He attributed the ignorance to the "long-standing neglect of nutrition in medical education and in health care delivery systems."

If such neglect of nutritional requirements is the case in hospitals staffed by multitudes of specialists armed with testing equipment, what must be happening in the offices of overworked doctors across the land?

A diabetic man of twenty-four who had been dependent upon insulin since the age of nine developed nephrotic syndrome, peripheral neuropathy, and muscular atrophy, the *Nutrition Today* article notes. After being released from the hospital he stayed in bed at home for two months, eating a poor diet with no vitamin supplement. He was later admitted to the hospital with extensive skin lesions and other clinical features revealing pellagra.

"A vitamin supplement," Dr. Butterworth stated, "and better diet could have improved the patient's sense of well being and eliminated the need for hospitalization."

Based on his studies Dr. Butterworth concluded: "We believe this preliminary analysis indicates an urgent need for a nutrition survey on a statistically adequate national sample of hospitalized patients.... There is every justification, and an urgent need, for ... revisions to be made without delay. Readers of *Nutrition Today* who are affiliated with a hospital are encouraged to look at the nutritional practices in their institutions. They shouldn't be surprised to find a skeleton behind the first door they open."

Behind the swinging doors

A two-year study in the mid-1970s by U.S. surgeons on the quality of their own work shows that nearly half the complications were preventable. So were 85 of the 245 surgical deaths investigated.

The Study of Surgical Services for the United States, a $1.5 million undertaking sponsored by the American College of Surgeons and the American Surgical Association, inspected the details of 1,696 deaths or complications associated with surgical procedures on 1,493 patients in ninety-five hospitals of seven states.

The January 26, 1976, issue of *Medical World News* states that an impressive 796 (47 percent) of the 1,696 incidents were assessed as preventable and 900 as nonpreventable by the cooperating hospitals.

You cannot control the surgical knife, but you can increase the chances of recovery in another way, as the following section suggests.

Helps for healing

If a hospital experience is looming on your horizon, prepare yourself for several weeks beforehand. Start early to fortify yourself for the ordeal by building up your health.

We suggest that you select foods loaded with protein to strengthen each organ with a good base on which to build. Your body can't store enough protein to last throughout your hospitalization, but you will be better off entering with a body fortified with excessive protein than with a body deficient in the substance of life.

The ideal breakfast offers one third the daily protein needs of the body. Protein eaten at sunup is more easily utilized by the body than protein eaten in the evening. If you choose cereal also, eat French toast or a cheese omelet. Wheat germ sprinkled over such a breakfast gives it additional protein power. Breakfast milk should be fortified with powdered milk for extra protein.

In the large hospital of a major American urban area an

attending physician remarked one day how extraordinary it was that a patient who had been burned severely was healing so rapidly. What the physician didn't know was that friends of the patient had watched for times when the nurses were out of the room. Then quickly they would break open capsules of vitamin E and spread it over the burn wounds externally. When the nurse inspected the wound the area looked just as it might from normal secretion. The vitamin E did its work so well that no scar from the serious burn remained. The physician was later let in on the secret. He instituted a policy of similar treatment for all burn patients admitted to the hospital.

A nutritionist crusader regularly smuggled vitamins and "live" food into hospitals for patients among his circle of friends. Patients he visited complained that it was nearly impossible to convince the reluctant nurses that recuperating patients needed extra protein and food supplements. He found also that special diets other than those for diabetes and obesity practically do not exist in hospitals.

Medical institutions have generally been slow to catch on to the blessings of nutrition in curing the sick. Take a survey in your area. You will understand the predicament more clearly and be able to help improve the situation.

A friend of ours recently arranged for rhinoplasty (corrective nasal surgery) to remedy injuries suffered in an accident. Before the operation he fortified himself with a high-protein diet and vitamin/mineral supplements.

Our friend was rewarded by exclamations of surprise when the surgeon removed the bandages and made his first inspection. There had been far less bruising than normal. In the following days not one nosebleed occurred. The surgeon said it was one of the cleanest cases he had ever seen—attributable, we think, to the preoperative nutrition observed by our friend.

Nutrition and the troops

A special study carried out among the U.S. Armed Forces by the National Academy of Sciences, National Research Council, found that therapeutic nutrition dramatically increased the number of soldiers saved in battle. The mortality rates from combat injuries in World War II were about half those of World War I. One of the main reasons was the military's attention to the nutritional requirements of patients.

"The state of nutrition affects the resistance of the individual to disease and the capacity of the tissue for repair," stated a council report. Since soldiers must be kept at peak efficiency and, when injured, returned to active duty as quickly as possible, long periods of convalescence create liabilities in logistics.

The government report found that "medical school curricula are preoccupied with diagnoses and specific therapy. Little time and attention are directed toward the nutritional aspect of therapeutics."

The medical graduate, the report stated, "is expected to learn this aspect during his internship and residency. The hospital attending physician whose responsibility it is to teach the house staff, interested as he is in the intellectual challenge of diagnosis, not infrequently neglects the adequacy of the patient's diet. The house officer, frequently identifying himself with his chief, also tends to relegate this aspect of the patient's care to the nurses and dieticians. He thereby neglects not only the patient but also his own training. It is not sufficient to bring technical and training manuals up to date. The medical corps must educate its personnel in the daily use of the manuals and in the application of the newer knowledge of nutrition."

The Research Council of the National Academy of Sciences drew an analogy between nutrition and optimum efficiency:

"Good nutrition is an essential element in good health. It is important for normal organ development and function, for normal growth of the organism as a whole, for optimum efficiency, for maximal resistance to infection, and for the ability to combat successfully disease and injury."

The report by the prestigious committee stated: "A well defined nutritional program can be of assistance in increasing the speed of convalescence and the return of a casualty to full active duty. The success of such a program demands aggressiveness in execution. The responsibility for the execution rests not only on the nurse and hospital corpsman but directly on the ward officer, the chief of service and the commanding officer."

The findings of the military report can be applied also to the layman's experience in the hospital. The better fortified a patient is when he goes into the hospital, the more quickly he is released. Patients who have to undergo surgery should receive abundant protein both preoperatively and postoperatively. About 150 grams per day are indicated.

Hospital malnutrition. The two words should never have to appear next to each other. Your concern and action can help change the picture, beginning in your local community and spreading across the nation.

Hospital survival kit

It is a proven fact that patients recover from surgery or serious disease more rapidly when they are fortified with extra doses of vitamins and minerals.

Here is how you, or a loved one, can hasten the exit from a bed of pain:

1. Stock a supply of multiple vitamin-mineral tablets in your personal belongings. If your doctor has not prescribed a supplement, tell him you plan to continue your

daily habit of food supplements during your hospital stay because they are vitally important to your recovery. If he objects, you can do one of two things: find an enlightened doctor; or keep cool, and smuggle supplements into the hospital or have your family bring them to you. The evidence that they will speed your recovery is overwhelming.

2. When selecting your menu, order:
• Fresh fruits and fresh green salads as much as possible (unless restricted by your doctor).
• Turkey, chicken, fish, lean beef, cheese, eggs, or soybean products (at least one of these protein foods at each meal).
• Baked potatoes instead of mashed or fried (most cooked vegetables are water-logged and a nutritional fiasco. Ask if you can order cottage cheese or another salad in place of the cooked vegetable.
• Yogurt for dessert (especially important if you've been taking an antibiotic).
• Whole-wheat bread and pat of butter.

3. Add protein powder to the milk or juices. We highly recommend a "Serenity Cocktail" developed by Mrs. Gladys Lindberg which contains all the essential amino acids. It is abundant in protein, calcium, and phosphorus. This may be ordered through the Lindberg Nutrition Service in Los Angeles, California.

4. Refrain from all sugar and chocolate served from the hospital kitchen or given as gifts from well-meaning but thoughtless visitors.

5. Abstain from caffeine drinks including coffee, tea, chocolate, and colas. Request juice or milk. Have your family bring you herbal tea bags and blackstrap molasses to add to milk.

6. Saturate your mind with the comfort available from the Holy Scriptures.

7. Maintain an optimistic outlook. Inner peace and serenity contribute to the healing process.

(Suggestion: Have a loved one phone the hospital in advance and inquire about their food. Have an idea of what you face nutritionally so you can be prepared. If you are going to pay $100 plus per day for hospital care, you have a right to know what you will eat.)

THINGS TO DO

1. Before a hospital experience, fortify the body with high-protein foods.

2. Also eat foods high in vitamins A and C so your body will be equipped to fight the effects of stress and possible infection.

3. Pack food supplements among your personal belongings.

4. Order wisely from the hospital menu while recuperating.

5. Use the hospital survival kit suggested in this chapter for yourself and loved ones.

Kefir

Kefir is a healing cultured milk drink that is thick like buttermilk and tastes like yogurt. Flavored with natural sweeteners, it is a zesty anytime drink that will delight your taste buds. It is a favorite substitute for yogurt.

Kefir is made from whole pasteurized milk by adding friendly beneficial bacteria, containing Lactobacillus Caucasicus of the Lactobacillus Acidophilus family and Lactobacillus Bulgaricus.

Why should you drink kefir? Some think the word came from *keif*, a Turkish word meaning "good feeling." And kefir lives up to its name.

It stimulates the flow of digestive juices in the gastrointestinal tract and serves as an excellent postoperative food to restore peristalsis, which often ceases in abdominal operations.

The drink is an excellent natural laxative used to eliminate constipation. It puts back good bacteria which antibiotics remove, fortifying the body against pathogenic organisms.

You can make it in your home. Start with a supply of fresh kefir grains placed in whole or skim milk. Stir, cover, then permit the mixture to stay at room temperature (65° to 75° F.) for two to three days. Afterward the milk will be thick. Pour it through a sieve. What drops through the sieve is Kefir. The curd that remains in the sieve is the active Kefir grains which can be used over again.

Yogurt

One of the finest foods available is also one of the least understood in America. Yogurt is a cultured milk food which has a fascinating ability to coax good health from the body. It's not just another form of milk.

Fermented milk products provide more food value than is available in sweet milk. During the culturing of cows' milk which changes it into yogurt, the biological value of the protein increases. The lactose of milk is converted into lactic acid, which is good news for your digestion. Yogurt offers your body calcium and phosphorus in a more easily assimilated form.

What else can the snow-white food provide? Yogurt hinders the growth of, or kills, pathogenic organisms responsible for illness and death in humans and animals. Many pathogens, like those causing dysentery, cannot thrive in an acid medium such as lactic acid.

Yogurt controls diarrhea in newborn infants and in young children. Fermented yogurt, rather than sweet milk fresh from the cow, is preferred for weaning infants in the Soviet Union. Properties of yogurt—acidophilus and bulgaricus—seem to act as intestinal antibiotics, preventing illness and making the sick well. An eight-ounce jar of yogurt has an antibiotic value equivalent to 14 units of penicillin! Antibiotic drugs destroy normal intestinal flora resulting in constipation or diarrhea; yogurt restores the balance and lets the body heal itself.

If eating it straight is not to your liking, flavor with fruit or honey. Yogurt can keep you well stocked in friendly flora that will do battle against the onslaught of germs your body faces daily.

Homemade Yogurt

Any variety of milk may be used—milk from a cow, goat, sheep, or even soybean milk. Milk may be fresh, whole, or nonfat, but not canned.

Starters:

- Use a fresh commercial starter of Lactobacillus Bulgaricus culture.

    Or

- Use a high-grade unflavored commercial yogurt made with Lactobacillus Bulgaricus culture.

Choice of recipes:

1 quart fresh milk
¼ cup dry milk
1 Tbsp. commercial starter

Or

1 quart fresh milk
¼ cup dry milk
¼ cup fresh commercial yogurt

Blend liquid and dry milk together. Heat until hot, then

allow milk to cool to approximately 110° F. (Test the milk on your wrist or use a kitchen thermometer.) Add the starter and stir well. Scald a jar or custard cups so they will be clean and warm. Pour yogurt into these containers for the incubation period. Commercial yogurt makers are convenient but not necessary. Cover the containers with lids or foil and place in warm place. The temperature around yogurt while it is culturing should be about 107° and no higher than 112°. If the milk temperature is too hot, the yogurt-making bacteria will be destroyed.

For instance, custard cups could be placed in electric skillet with warm 112° water, covered, and allowed to stand for 2-4 hours until thick. If using a large jar, wrap in towel and place in warm oven. Permit heated oven to cool to about 100°. Or place jar near pilot light heat. A friend of ours uses large jars in a covered styrofoam chest kept heated by warm water surrounding the jars.

Refrigerate finished yogurt and use within a week. The finished product will thicken when chilled. We suggest you flavor the yogurt at the time of serving and not the entire batch as it is ready. You cannot use flavored yogurt for culturing a new batch.

Serve yogurt with sliced fresh fruit, or as a honey sundae with nuts. Use for dressings, soups, baked potatoes, etc.

CHAPTER TWELVE

Good Health Is a Habit

Habit is stronger than nature.—Quintus Curtius Rufus

If the fat is indeed in your head, as Charlie Shedd proves in his book by that title, obese human beings literally dig their graves with their teeth.

If proper exercise banishes fatigue, burns food more efficiently, and helps tune up your priceless machine, many people are asking for health problems by refusing to get enough of it.

If stress from lack of sleep is the quickest way to mental breakdown, robbing the body of proper rest is short-sighted.

Observe the nutritional trio of proper food, exercise, and rest. Are you giving equal attention to each?

What you don't know can *hurt you*

Providing all the proteins, vitamins, minerals, carbohydrates, fats, and water your body needs is the best way to keep it free from disease and to fortify it against stress. All these elements are found in food. A good diet has various combinations. Not all are present in any single food. You may need vitamin-mineral supplements.

The blessings of optimum nutrition through good eating habits is the theme of this book. Your own eating habits may have been needlessly complicated by pressure to conform to a multitude of fad diets. Some nutritional overlap occurs, except in foods with empty calories, so relax. Make eating enjoyable as well as purposeful.

Eat an abundance of "live" (raw) foods such as salads, fresh fruits, and fresh vegetables. If you do cook vegetables such as carrots, which release more carotene and vitamin A after cooking, use low heat with little or no water to drain off later.

Run for your life

A professor in Chicago used to say, "When I get the feeling that I need exercise I lie down until the feeling goes away." Everyone laughed when he said it. A clever line, indeed, but an unfortunate practice because it was literally true. Our friend later paid a heavy price for his excesses.

To look your best, to feel your best, and to be able to do your best you must exercise regularly. That is required by man's nature, and modern technology can't change it.

When the physical activity required of you by your job and other duties falls below the level necessary to support good health, you must supplement it with planned activity. Your sense of well being, your ability to perform, and even your survival depend upon it.

The President's Council on Physical Fitness and Sports has published a survey showing that 45 percent of all adult Americans (roughly 49 million of the 109 million total) do not engage in physical activity for the purpose of exercise; only 55 percent of American men and women do any exercise at all, but 57 percent say they believe they get enough exercise.

One of the most popular exercise programs which has endured the test of critics and disciples has been a technique called "aerobics." In a book by that name, Kenneth H. Cooper, M.D., outlined for the Air Force an approach to exercise which introduced no new exercises but rather a system of measuring the value of old ones. The theme of the book could be stated in three words: "Get your oxygen!"[1] Thus a person who swims, runs, or rides a bicycle hard to develop his wind has it hands down over a weight lifter or a fan of isometrics who exercises to develop skeletal muscles.

The amount of exercise needed varies from one individual to another. From thirty to sixty minutes a day is recommended. The way you exercise is just as important as how often it is done. For optimum benefit, physical activity must be vigorous enough to give a tonic effect. In other words, the individual must work hard enough to breathe heavily and "break a sweat."

Persons unfamiliar with the principles of exercise seldom work hard enough or long enough to improve circulatory and respiratory performance or to strengthen muscles. One reason for this is that many of our more popular and enjoyable participatory sports are not taxing enough for fitness purposes. They make a contribution but should be supplemented by an exercise regimen.

Exercise will help your body assimilate the proper nutrition you have pledged to give it. Hand in hand, exercise and nutrition offer big rewards to the consistent patron.

Before you begin

Before beginning any exercise program, it is advisable to have a medical checkup. If you have not had an examination in the past year, if you are past thirty, if you are over-weight, or if you have a history of high blood pressure or heart trouble, such an examination may help you to avoid extremely serious consequences.

Exercise capacity varies widely among individuals, even when they are similar in age and physical build. That's why your program should be based on your personal test re-sults, rather than on what someone else is doing, or on what you think you should be able to do. Only as your body is properly exercised can it assimilate the good nutrition that you give it.

"Good night"

Just because you may have important work to do, this doesn't mean that the Creator is going to suspend the laws of sleep by which we all must live. Humbling as it is, we all have to prostrate ourselves at the end of the day and "die." Thus the body is restored and refreshed for another sun-rise.

Dr. Robert Smith, Professor of Philosophy at Bethel Col-lege, St. Paul, Minnesota, said in his lecture circuit that he finds "numerous family quarrels, broken homes and lack of joy in the lives of people who somehow think they are angels and don't need to be concerned about sleep."

Writing in the July 1974 *Worldwide Impact* magazine, he tells of a young husband who sought the counsel of a bril-liant internist. "Doc," the young man complained, "I just don't know what's the matter with me. My wife says that I'm as sour as a bear with a thorn in its paw."

He told the doctor about some of the physical aches and pains that he was having and asked him to check him over thoroughly.

"I'm just dogging it," the young man said.

The doctor listened carefully. *All he needs is sleep,* he said to himself. *But he won't accept my advice if I tell him just to go home and go to bed.* So he said to his patient, "Next week we will give you all the tests, but it is very expensive and I don't want to put any more expense on you than I have to. So, before we start the tests, I want you to be well rested. To-night I want you to go home and get twelve hours' sleep. And I want you to have twelve hours of sleep tomorrow, Wednesday, and Thursday. Then call me on Friday."

The young man immediately thought of a variety of church meetings he had to attend, but finally agreed to cooperate. On Friday the call came. "Man, I haven't felt so good in fifteen years," he told his doctor. "We don't need those tests."

Dr. Smith said he finds men and women at the university going without sleep for twelve hours, and then twenty-four ... thirty-six ... forty-eight ... and seventy-two! Very soon, he said, they begin to reveal symptoms of schizophrenia and paranoia. The students become edgy, irritable, and can't get along with people. Dr. Smith observed that they develop self-centeredness and gloomy countenances— primarily because they simply haven't given their bodies rest.

One man's meat...

Just for fun, and as a bit of diversion, we stopped writing at this point and took pad and pencil for a survey. We walked through our cabin at Hume Lake, California, where our grandmother, aunt, nephews, and sons had gathered for a vacation. "Off the top of your head," we asked each one, "what's your advice for keeping healthy?"

The answers are recorded just as they were given by our enthusiastic family:

Grandmother: "Bathe every day, for cleanliness is next to godliness."

Aunt Jo: "Drink lots of water."

Nephew Bruce: "Get out on the surf at least once a day."
Nephew Bryan: "Don't get behind in your homework."
Son Randy: "Read the Bible and pray."
Son Rusty: "Goals. Keep a lot of goals out there to get you going."

Well, fitness is a lot of things, to be sure. And perhaps no one in our family mentioned proper rest, nutrition, and exercise because they take them for granted. Our television set is unplugged by unanimous vote. We keep projects humming and spread the board with a variety of foods as fresh as we can get them. As for sleep, we parents try to set an example in this area and children quite naturally follow after.

It's your move

Your fitness for enjoyable living implies freedom from disease ... strength and to spare for work and play ... a good emotional reserve to answer stress ... mental development to be all you can be in the profession you've chosen.

Although your ultimate fitness depends largely upon the body you inherited, you can reach your top limits by discipline in practicing health habits. Your body is responsive to training; it operates under a wide safety margin and is strikingly resistant to strain.

Remember: Nothing in your life is unaffected by nutrition. Without it you can't think; without it you can't work; without it you can't play; without it you can't love God, your neighbor, or yourself as you should.

The next move is up to you.

> Don't you know that you yourselves are God's temple and that God's Spirit lives in you? If anyone destroys God's temple, God will destroy him, for God's temple is sacred, and you are that temple.
> —1 Corinthians 3:16, 17 (New International Version)

DECLARATION OF DEPENDENCE

I'll join the nutrition revolution.

Recognizing my responsibility to care for the body which God has given me, I hereby determine as much as possible to avoid foods that kill in favor of foods that heal, in order to stay alive and vibrant on planet earth all the days of my life, so help me God.

Signed _____

A Salute to the Serious

For those who recognize their responsibility to keep their marvelous bodies running at peak efficiency, here is additional information concerning:
1. Priority foods
2. Go-easy foods
3. Foods to forget
Included also are tips on:
1. Cooking fresh vegetables
    a. Waterless technique
    b. Steaming technique
    c. Stir-fry technique
2. Cooking fresh meat
3. Benefits of fiber
    a. Sources
    b. Recipes
4. Kitchen tools and utensils
    a. Basic hardware
    b. Handy measurements

Priority Foods

Alfalfa (in tablet form)

This food is loaded with enormous amounts of vitamins, is high in minerals and protein, and is filled with essential amino acids.

Avocado

This delectable food offers iron, calcium, phosphorus, magnesium, copper, manganese, potassium, sodium, vitamins A, B_1, B_2, niacin, and vitamin C. A whole avocado has beneficial fiber and four grams of protein. It contains hardly any sugar or starch. The oil in the avocado has a high percentage of polyunsaturated fatty acids. It is a true wonder food that we should eat generously. Don't worry about the calories. The body burns vegetable oils easily.

Beans

Soybeans are superior, but all beans are a fine source of protein. Soybean products such as soy flour, soy powder, soy milk, and soy grits are some of the most valuable sources of protein.

Blackstrap molasses

This is a food rich in potassium, calcium, phosphorus, iron, and the B vitamins (B_1, B_2, B_3 and B_6). It's an acceptable sweetener but does not contain sugar.

Brewer's yeast

This is an astonishingly nutritious substance. It has nineteen amino acids, all of the B vitamins, and a veritable dictionary of coveted elements. Get it! You won't regret it.

Breads

Whole-grain bread gives you the much-needed B vitamins, trace minerals, and fiber. White bread has been depleted of B vitamins and fiber necessary to a good diet.

Carob

See amplification on page 175.

Cheeses

Natural cheese is high in minerals and protein. Cottage cheese, especially, is an excellent source of protein.

Cereals

Whole-grain (such as seven-grain) cereals, oatmeal, soy grits, Scotch oats, corn, rice, whole-wheat cereals, bran, granola, etc., are choice ingredients to an adequate diet.

Eggs

An egg is high in protein but low in fat. This nearly perfect food has selenium, zinc, phosphorus, calcium, sulphur, vitamin A, vitamin B_{12}, choline, tryptophan, pyridoxine (B_6), riboflavin (B_2), thiamine (B_1), folic acid, and pantothenic acid. Eggs are a perfect food premeasured and prepackaged. They contain the essential amino acids.

Fruits

Fresh fruit should be selected as often as possible. It is a good source of minerals, vitamins A and C.

Honey

See page 59.

Kefir

See chapter 11.

Liver

This meat is a marvelous food for various reasons: It is a complete protein containing all the essential amino acids. The iron content is high. It is also very high in vitamins A and C. Liver should be eaten at least once a week.

Milk powder

Milk in powdered form is one of the most concentrated and economic sources of a complete protein. There are two kinds of powdered milk that should be used. Following are the nonfat values:

⅔ cup noninstantized milk   35 grams of protein
⅔ cup instant milk   18 grams of protein

Measure for measure, the noninstant is 50 percent higher in protein.

The instant is what you buy in the supermarket under the names of Carnation, Sanalac, Jerseymaid, etc. The noninstant is available in health specialty stores. It is not only higher in protein value but has escaped the intense heat used in the other, heat which destroys valuable enzymes. Use much of the noninstantized milk as a boost to regular milk, cookies, meat loaf, etc. Our fudge recipes are made with this milk.

If you consume adequate amounts of milk, your body will be furnished with more protein of high biological value and more calcium and phosphorus than any other food the daily diet can supply.

Nuts

From the almond, king of nuts, to the lowly peanut, few sources of protein are more tasty, handy to eat, and healthful. The variety is almost endless. To be well digested, nuts must be eaten raw and chewed well. Roasted nuts, or nuts which have been dipped in hot fat or boiled, have lost their enzyme content. That is why nuts are often called the food that is difficult to digest. Eat them fresh from the shell in their natural state.

Seeds

The various edible seeds available to humans are the source for new plant life. They offer all the vitamins, minerals, proteins, fats, and carbohydrates required for sprouting and for the sprout's initial growth. The lowly sunflower seed offers an example. It has twice as much iron as raisins and abundant potassium which is linked to the health of nerves and muscles. Twenty-five percent of its weight is protein. It also has fiber which promotes the swift passage of wastes through the intestinal tract.

Sprouts

Closely aligned in value with seeds, sprouts are the most living food available. Vitamin and mineral content of seeds increases with the sprouting process. The recommended sprouts are alfalfa, Chinese cabbage, cress (pepper grass), foenugreek, special pea, lentil, mung bean, mustard, oat groats, pichi bean, porridge pea, radish, red clover, rye, soybean, sunflower, wheat, and Alaskan pea. Our boys enjoyed raising sprouts right in our kitchen with a plastic container and regular periods of watering.

Yogurt

See page 228.

Go-Easy Foods

Canned fruit. This inadequate food is overcooked and loaded with large amounts of sugar.

Canned vegetables. These are overcooked, over-salted, and may have harmful chemicals.

Cold cereals. Preservatives and sugar abound. Lack of trace minerals and fiber.

Macaroni. Starch equals sugar.

Noodles. Starch equals sugar.

Spaghetti. Starch equals sugar.

Fat meats. High in saturated fats.

Foods to Forget

All sugar and refined carbohydrates.

Sugar-laden pies, cakes, French pastries, donuts, cookies made with saturated fat (shortening).

Saturated fats like shortening, chocolate, coconut.

All cola drinks made with sugar and synthetic canned "fruit" drinks (buy pure fruit juices instead).

All processed and precooked frozen dinners and side dishes (too many chemicals).

Packaged meats that have the dangerous sodium nitrate and sodium nitrite chemicals (see section on chemical poisoning).

Coffee. If you are fond of it, as we are, switch to decaffeinated coffee and you'll feel better. Or switch to herbal tea for a hot drink. Get your pickup from protein snacks. Coffee robs your body of B vitamins.

Chocolate. It interferes with mineral utilization and is high in saturated fat.

White bread. It has lost the wheat germ containing protein, B vitamins, vitamin E, and fiber.

French fries. Many are presalted and cooked in oils that are not kept fresh. When fat is heated and reheated a chemical process takes place causing it to become carcinogenic. Fatty acids break down at high temperatures.

Candy. Even high-quality candy is devastating to the body—from the teeth to the pancreas.

Licorice. This substance can cause serious health problems. Symptoms of licorice poisoning are headaches, high blood pressure, heart palpitations, and weakness. (Report was given in *Medical Tribune.*)

Maraschino cherries. These are saturated with harmful dyes and preservatives.

Cooking Fresh Vegetables

"Cover with water; cook 20 minutes, then drain."

That simple statement, and others like it, have put oceans of nutrients into the sewer. It's tragic, but true. The cook of tomorrow will need to edit each recipe. Each time the word "drain" appears it should be edited out.

Nutrients in vegetables can be destroyed through oxidation, excessive heat, and water. We strongly recommend the scientific method of waterless cooking.

How you cook fresh vegetables depends largely upon the age, amount, and size of the pieces of each vegetable. The following tips should be observed in preparing all vegetables:

Vegetables need not be peeled unless the recipe calls for it. If vegetables must be peeled, peel carefully to avoid loss of the valuable minerals close to the skin.

Waterless technique

Place vegetables in utensil. Pan should be at least ⅔ full, preferably altogether full. Cover with cold water for a moment, then pour off quickly. The moisture that clings is sufficient for "waterless" cooking. Most vegetables contain enough natural water. If at first you're not sure of this technique, add 1 to 2 tablespoons of water until you perfect it. If using mature, starchy vegetables, more may be needed.

Cover utensil and place on medium heat. At the first sign of vapor, reduce heat to low. If it is necessary to test vegetables, raise edge of cover just enough to insert a fork. Cook until tender; season and serve.

Of course, dried fruits, rice, and soups need quantities of water for proper cooking. Here we're concerned with fresh vegetables. We usually don't recommend the cooking of fruits. It is necessary for babies and for special diets, but raw fruit is the best and most nutritious because we can have the benefit of more enzyme activity. Applesauce is a favorite at our house, but a raw apple is such a perfect package of goodness that we don't like to tamper with it too often.

Steaming technique

Steaming your vegetables over water is also an acceptable method and certainly is superior to water-logged vegetables. However, in our testing, steaming does not retain the flavor as well as waterless cooking. The only exception is corn on the cob.

Chinese stir-fry technique

Use a heavy skillet or wok pan. Add a little oil and stir constantly while frying the vegetable or meat. Vegetables remain crisp and nutritious with this method.

Time Chart for Vegetables

Four-Six Servings	*Minutes*
Asparagus	10 - 15
Beans, green cut	20 - 25
Beans, wax cut	20 - 25
Beans, green limas	20 - 30
Beets, whole	30 - 45
Broccoli	10 - 20
Brussels sprouts	10 - 20
Cabbage (shredded)	3 - 10
Carrots (sliced)	10 - 20
Carrots (whole)	15 - 25
Cauliflower broken into flowerets	8 - 15
Celery (1″ length)	10 - 20
Corn (frozen)	3 - 5
Onions, small whole	15 - 25
Parsnips, sliced	20 - 30
Peas	8 - 20
Potatoes, quartered	15 - 25
Potatoes, sweet, quartered	15 - 25
Rutabagas, cubed	20 - 30
Spinach	3 - 10
Squash, green summer	10 - 15
Squash, yellow crook neck	10 - 15
Squash, zucchini	10 - 15
Squash, winter, cubed	20 - 40
Tomatoes	7 - 15
Turnips	20 - 30

Cooking Meats
(pork ... beef ... veal ... poultry ... fish)

Low-temperature, top-of-stove roasting is the tasty, economical way to prepare meats. High heat toughens meat, drives out natural juices, and creates wasteful shrinkage. Low-temperature meat cooking retains flavorful juices, makes meats tasty and tender, and cuts shrinkage losses to a minimum.

Generally, frozen meats need not be thawed before cooking, but frozen meat does require more cooking time to allow for thawing. When meat is thawed before cooking, it should be in the refrigerator or at approximately 40° temperature. Higher temperatures during thawing increase shrinkage.

Four Methods

Braising

Place meat in utensil over medium heat. Add a small piece of fat if meat is lean. Brown thoroughly on all sides. Season. Place cover on the utensil. When vapors begin to rise from the cover, turn heat to low. Continue cooking until done.

Pan broiling

Place meat in skillet over medium heat and brown on both sides. Fat or water need not be added. Leave skillet uncovered. After browning meat, reduce heat to low and cook slowly. Pour off excess fat as it accumulates. Season and serve when done.

Sauteing

Place meat in skillet. Add a small amount of oil. Brown carefully over medium heat. Season and cook at low temperature until done. Turn occasionally. Do not cover. Serve as soon as done.

Roasting

For low-temperature stove-top roasting, place roast in dutch oven. Using medium heat, brown roast evenly on all sides. Season. Cover and reduce heat to low. For oven roasting, place meat fat side up in open roasting pan. Season and place in slow oven. Do not add water, cover, or baste. Continue cooking at recommended temperature until done.

Oven roasting at a very low temperature is most acceptable. The oven should be set at 150°-175°. A roast can cook unattended for about 8 hours if you like it rare. Cook for another hour if you like it well done. The meat roasted at this low temperature assures even cooking all the way through. It is not necessary to wait the usual 20 minutes before carving the roast, but it can be cut immediately. This method can be used for a rump roast, rolled beef roast, cross rib roast, or sirloin tip. The 8-hour figure is based on a 4-5 pound roast.

The California Beef Council has tested this method and has given its approval. The meat is safe cooked at this low temperature, but never lower than 150°. In fact, your oven may only have a setting for as low as 175°, and that is fine. Try this method and you'll enjoy the aroma filling the house for hours.

Benefits of Fiber

The nutritional qualities of food are most often described in terms of their protein, carbohydrates, fats, vitamins, and mineral content. The importance of fiber or roughage in the diet has been less frequently mentioned, although its value in promoting bowel regularity probably has been recognized through the ages.

Only plant sources provide fiber for our diet. Some foods which are high in fiber are blackberries, raspberries, dates, lima beans, black beans, whole wheat, and all bran.

The fiber absorbs many times its own weight in water, thus promoting softer stools. Good elimination helps the body to protect itself against many noninfectious diseases of the large intestine that are prevalent in our society, including cancer.

Many physicians—notably columnists and doctors who have the ability to popularize medical subjects in books—are giving more attention to fiber than ever. Studies show that obesity, diabetes, coronary heart disease, and certain bowel disorders are less prevalent in Africa than in North America and Western Europe. High fiber content in an African's diet seems to be one reason.

Keep in mind that dietary fiber is made up of many substances, and the composition differs in cereals, vegetables, fruits, and seeds. So a variety of plant foods is needed in our diets. This is another reason your choice of foods should be from a wide variety.

As a general rule, unrefined foods contain more roughage than refined foods because some fiber is usually removed in processing. By eating fiber-rich foods you increase the speed of food through the intestine and allow for less opportunity for constipation. In addition, fiber-rich food results in stools which are quite different both chemically and bacteriologically. Increased retention of the stool in the colon and the difference in chemical and bacterial composition may lead to local irritation of the cells of the colon, inviting cancer.

In the past years we haven't paid enough attention to the roughage in our diets. But because of its increasingly recognized importance, the nutrition spotlight is being focused on dietary fiber. The need for fiber now turns consumers' concern more than ever to the dangers of over-milled, overrefined, and highly processed food. The daily need for fiber is 5-6 grams.

Sources of Fiber

Fruits	*Grams*
Apples	1.5
Avocados (one half)	1.6
Banana (one)	.8
Blackberries (½ cup)	3.0
Blueberries (½ cup)	1.1
Dates, pitted (½ cup)	2.1
Honeydew melon (2″ × 6″ slice)	.8
Orange (1 medium)	.8
Prunes (½ cup)	1.2
Raspberries, black (½ cup)	3.8
Raspberries, red (½ cup)	2.0
Strawberries (½ cup)	1.0

Vegetables	
Asparagus (5 spears)	.5
Beans, green (½ cup)	.6
Beet greens (½ cup)	1.1
Broccoli (½ cup)	1.1
Brussels sprouts (½ cup)	1.1
Cucumber (1 med.)	1.7
Eggplant (½ cup)	.9
Okra (½ cup)	.8
Peas (½ cup)	1.6
Sweet peppers (½ cup)	1.0
Potatoes (baked 1)	.7
Potatoes (mashed ½ cup)	.5
Rutabagas (½ cup)	1.1
Squash, acorn (½ cup)	1.6
Sweet potato (1 med.)	1.5
Tomato (1 med.)	.8

Legumes & beans	
Black beans (1 cup cooked)	3.0
Chick peas (1 cup cooked)	2.5
Kidney beans (1 cup cooked)	2.3

Lima beans (1 cup cooked) 2.9
Pinto beans (1 cup cooked) 2.3

Misc.
Hamburgers (McDonald's)
   1 Big Mac 9
   1 Hamburger 5
   Quarter Pounder 6
The pickle, lettuce, and sesame seeds on the bun bring up
the fiber content surprisingly.

Grains
Bread (1 slice)
   pumpernickel 4
   whole-wheat 4
   white 1
   rye 1

Cereals
Oatmeal 4
Wheatena 5

Cereals ready to eat
All-Bran 2.1
Bran Buds 2.0
Bran Flakes 1.0
Grape-Nuts (¼ cup) 4
Raisin Bran (½ cup) 9
Total (1 cup) 4
Wheat Chex 8

Cornmeal flour (1 cup)
All purpose (1 cup unsifted) 2
Whole-wheat (1 cup unsifted) 2.8

Rice
Brown (½ cup cooked) 2
White (½ cup cooked) 1

Waffle
One 8" ....trace

Our Favorite Granola

7 cups rolled oats,
  uncooked (Quakers 1 lb.
  2 oz. size)
1 cup sunflower seeds,
  crushed in blender
½ cup sesame seeds,
  crushed in blender
1 cup almonds (or pecans,
  cashews, peanuts, or
  walnuts). Crush in
  plastic bag with rolling
  pin.

1 cup unprocessed bran
  flakes*
¼ cup soy granules
  (lecithin)
1 tsp. iodized salt
1 cup soy oil
1 cup pure honey
1 Tbsp. vanilla

Heat oats in large baking pan, with enough room to stir (suggest 18" × 12" size). Bake for 10 minutes in preheated 325° oven. Remove pan from oven and add seeds, nuts, bran, lecithin, and salt. Mix well. Pour oil, honey, and vanilla over dry ingredients and stir until blended. Return to oven and reduce heat to 300°. Bake for another 25-30 minutes, stirring often to keep oats from scorching. Cool. Crumble and store in airtight container.

  At serving time sprinkle with:
wheat germ (keep in
  refrigerator as it
  becomes rancid)
moist raisins or
chopped prunes or
chopped apple or
sliced banana

*Eliminate bran if allergic to wheat.

Mom Rohrer's Chicken Corn Soup

1 chicken, a 3-4 lb. hen cut up
3 quarts of cold water
1 onion, chopped
½ cup chopped celery and leaves
10 ears fresh corn (or frozen)
salt and pepper
2 cooked eggs, chopped

Cook chicken slowly with water, onion, and celery. Simmer until tender, adding salt 30 minutes before it is done. Remove chicken and strain broth through a fine sieve. Take meat from bones and chop fine and return to broth. Cut the corn from the cob and add to soup. Season with salt and pepper and simmer for several more minutes. Just before serving add the chopped eggs. Serves 6.

Baby Lima Bean Soup

1 lb. baby lima beans
7 cups cold water
1 grated carrot
½ onion, grated
2 Tbsp. chopped fresh cilantro
1 Tbsp. fresh or home-dried celery leaves
1 Tbsp. fresh parsley, chopped or dried
1 clove garlic, grated or put through press
salt and pepper to taste

Soak beans in water overnight. Do not drain. Add vegetables and seasonings. Cook all ingredients together for one hour or until tender. Delicious served with corn bread and coleslaw.

Cabbage for the King

4 cups finely shredded
  cabbage (approx.
  one-half head)
½ cup thinly sliced celery
½ cup chopped cucumber
2 Tbsp. diced green
  pepper
2 Tbsp. diced green
  onions
1 Tbsp. minced parsley
½ or 1 avocado

Dressing:
¼ cup mayonnaise
¼ cup sour cream
½ tsp. salt
1 Tbsp. lemon juice or
  vinegar
dash of artificial sweetener
dash of pepper
dash of paprika

Have all the vegetables well chilled before preparing. Mix in a large mixing bowl together. Prepare the dressing and toss with the salad mixings. Garnish with avocado slices. The dressing may be thinned with cream or fruit juice if preferred.

Seven Cylinder Salad

1. 1 lb. fresh carrots,
   cooked
2. 1 lb. fresh string beans,
   cooked
3. ½ lb. fresh peas,
   cooked
4. ½ lb. baby limas,
   cooked
5. ½ lb. kidney beans,
   cooked
6. 1 onion diced fine
7. 1 green pepper, diced

Dressing:
½ cup mayonnaise
1 cup sour cream
3 Tbsp. lemon juice or
  vinegar
2 Tbsp. honey or 1 Tbsp.
  artificial sweetener
1 tsp. salt
¼ to ½ tsp. dill weed

Cook vegetables, chill and mix together. Add dressing and toss until well marinated. Serve on a crisp lettuce leaf and garnish with hard-cooked eggs or pickled beets or both.

Tabbouli (Bulgur Wheat Salad*)

1 medium onion	2 tsp. fresh or dried mint
½ cup olive oil	1 cup *fine-grain* bulgur wheat
2 tomatoes, peeled & chopped	½ cup fresh parsley, minced
2 lemons, juiced	½ red onion, minced
½ cup tomato sauce	2 Tbsp. green bell pepper, minced
1 tsp. salt	3 green onions, minced
¼ tsp. pepper	

Sauté onion in olive oil. When onion is soft add one tomato, sauteing until onion is golden. Add lemon juice, tomato sauce, salt, pepper, and mint. Heat and remove from stove. Add bulgur wheat and let stand until all the juices are absorbed and the bulgur is fluffy. Refrigerate overnight. Add chopped parsley, bell pepper, red onion, and green onions. Dice remaining tomato and mix all together. Keep chilled until ready to serve. (If using coarse bulgur cook for 30-35 minutes before blending with other ingredients.) Serves 4 or 5. Recipe easily doubled.

*This delicious recipe was introduced to us by Adele Hopper of Fresno, Calif.

Orange Pecan Bread

2 eggs, beaten	2 tsp. baking powder
1 cup honey	¾ tsp. salt
3 Tbsp. vegetable oil	½ tsp. coriander
1 cup orange juice	1 cup whole bran
1 cup unbleached flour	1 cup finely chopped pecans
1 cup whole-wheat flour	

In a mixing bowl beat the eggs until frothy. Add the honey, oil, and orange juice, blending well. Sift all dry ingredients onto the liquids and blend. Stir in bran until moist. Fold in the pecans and pour batter into a buttered 9″ × 5″ loaf pan. Bake in a moderate 350° oven for 1 hour or until toothpick comes out clean. Makes one loaf.

Ranch Style Whole-Wheat Bread

½ cup warm water
2¼ cups milk
1 Tbsp. butter
⅓ cup honey
2 tsp. salt
2 pkgs. dry yeast

5¾ to 6 cups unsifted
  whole-wheat flour
¾ cup wheat kernels,
  ground in blender or
  coffee grinder
  (optional)

Combine water, milk, butter, honey, and salt in a 3-quart saucepan. Heat gently just to lukewarm. Dissolve the yeast in the liquid and allow to set until small bubbles begin to form, about 10 minutes. Stir in the flour until blended, and then stir in the ground wheat kernels. Knead until thoroughly mixed; set into a well-oiled bowl; flip over to coat top with oil and let rise 15-20 minutes, or until almost double in bulk. Turn dough out on a floured pastry cloth and knead 8-10 minutes until dough feels smooth and elastic. Divide dough into two equal pieces. Shape each piece into a loaf shape by rolling dough into an 8″ × 10″ rectangle. Break all gas bubbles. Beginning with upper 8-inch side, roll toward you, seal ends, and fold under, being careful not to tear dough. Place in two well-greased loaf pans 4½″ × 8½″. Let rise until dough is 1 inch higher than top of pan. Bake at 375° for 45 minutes or until done.

Variations:

Omit wheat kernels and add ½ cup nuts or dried, chopped fruits; or substitute coconut milk for cow's milk and add ½ cup grated coconut.

We thank home economist Libby Lafferty for this contribution. She is the instructor for the telecourse "Foods for the Modern Family" in Los Angeles.

Honey Bran Bars

Crust
½ cup butter
1 cup unbleached flour
⅓ cup fresh bran flakes
3 Tbsp. cold water
Filling
½ cup butter
1 cup water
1 cup unbleached flour

¼ teaspoon salt
3 eggs
½ cup honey
1 tsp. lemon juice
1 tsp. grated lemon rind
1 cup pecans, crushed in plastic bag with rolling pin

Cut butter into flour with pastry blender until crumbly. Stir in bran flakes. Sprinkle water over mixture and mix into a dough. Press the dough onto bottom of a buttered 13″ × 9″ pan.

In small saucepan melt butter with the water. Bring to a rolling boil and stir in flour and salt quickly. Cook over medium heat, blending well until mixture becomes stiff, about 1 minute. Remove from heat and beat in eggs one at a time, beating until smooth. Add honey, juice, and rind. Spread this batter over crust. Bake in 400° oven for 25 minutes. Remove and sprinkle with pecans; return to oven and bake 10 minutes more. Cool and cut into bars. Makes about 36.

Kitchen Tools and Utensils

Basic hardware for food preparation

3 mixing bowls (1 pint, 1 quart, 3 quart)
Small cutting board
1 slicing knife
1 3-inch paring knife
1 7-inch utility knife
1 butcher knife, 8-inch blade
1 peeler

1 pancake turner
pastry blender
flour sifter
rolling pin
1 spatula, 7-inch blade
1 rubber bowl scraper
wooden spoons, set of three
1 large cake-cooling rack
4 refrigerator storage dishes
1 metal mixing spoon
1 fork, 2 tines, long handle
combined grater and shredder
eggbeater
can opener
juicer
bottle or jar opener
colander or strainer
6-inch sieve
potato masher
vegetable brush
sink strainer
kitchen shears

For top-of-range cooking

1 double boiler, 1½ quart (designed so each section can be
   used separately on top of range)
1 saucepan, 1-quart with lid tight enough to cook waterless
1 saucepan, 3-quart with lid tight enough to cook waterless
1 kettle or dutch oven, 6-quart with tight lid
1 frypan, 8-inch omelet style
1 frypan, 12-inch
   Stainless steel Farberware and Ekco Flint cookware are
available in department stores. They meet standards for
waterless cooking. Vapor-seal covers are imperative.

For the oven

2 range-to-table casseroles with lids, 1-quart and 2-quart
2 6-cup muffin pans
2 layer cake pans, 8″ × 1½″
1 9-inch square pan
1 pie pan, 9-inch
1 loaf pan
1 9″ × 13″ baking dish
utility pan with rack
6 custard cups

For accurate measuring

1 set measuring spoons
1 set dry measures (¼, ⅓, ½, and 1 cup)
1 quart liquid measure
1 cup liquid measure

Appliances

blender
food grinder
electric mixer
electric skillet
slow cooker or crock pot
tea kettle
timer
toaster

Handy Measurement Chart

3 tsp. = 1 Tbsp.
2 Tbsp. = ⅛ cup
4 Tbsp. = ¼ cup
8 Tbsp. = ½ cup
12 Tbsp. = ¾ cup
16 Tbsp. = 1 cup
5 Tbsp. + 1 tsp. = ⅓ cup

4 oz. = ½ cup
8 oz. = 1 cup
16 oz. = 1 lb.
1 oz. = 2 Tbsp. fat or liquid
2 cups fat = 1 lb.
2 cups = 1 pt.
2 cups sugar = 1 lb.
⅝ cup = ½ cup + 2 Tbsp.
⅞ cup = ¾ cup + 2 Tbsp.
1 lb. butter = 2 cups or 4 sticks
2 pts. = 1 qt.
1 qt. = 4 cups
A few grains = less than ⅛ tsp.
Pinch = as much as can be taken between tip of finger and
    thumb
Speck = less than ⅛ tsp.

Table of Measurements

One gram equals 1000 milligrams or 15½ grains.
One mg. equals 1000 micrograms.
One gamma is the same as one microgram.
One mg. of vitamin C equals 20 USP units.
One milligram of vitamin B_1 equals 333 USP units.
One lb. equals 7000 grains.
One fluid ounce equals 29,573 cc.
One liter equals 1.0567 quarts.
30 grams equals 1 ounce.
64 mg. equals 1 grain.
452 gm. equals 1 lb.
1 tsp. yeast equals 4 gm.
6 tsp. equals 1 fluid ounce.

How the Average Shopper Spends a $20 Bill

FOOD

Fresh meat	$ 3.98
Produce	2.19
Dairy products	1.29
Baked goods & snacks	1.14
Misc. edibles	1.07
Frozen foods	1.06
Fresh poultry	.57
Coffee, tea	.52
Cereals, rice	.27
Dried fruits, vegetables, milk	.22
Canned Foods:	
Vegetables	.28
Meat & poultry	.22
Fruits	.18
Juices, drinks	.18
Seafood	.13
Soups	.12
Milk	.05
Fresh fish	.14
Sugar	.15
Macaroni, spaghetti, noodles	.09
Baby foods (excluding cereals)	.09
Jams, jellies, preserves	.07
Puddings	.03
TOTAL	$14.04

NONFOOD

Beer	$ .91
Misc. merchandise	.86
Health, beauty aids (non-Rx)	.76
Tobacco products	.75

Soft drinks	.45
Soaps, detergents, laundry	.43
Paper goods	.42
Other household products	.37
Pet foods	.27
Candy	.20
Housewares	.19
Groceries (not classified elsewhere)	.14
Wine, distilled spirits	.13
Prescriptions	.08
TOTAL	5.96
	$20.00

(Adapted from the 1974 "Supermarketing" consumer expenditure study)

FOOTNOTES

PREFACE
[1]Alan H. Nittler, *A New Breed of Doctor* (New York: Pyramid Books, 1972), p. xiii.

CHAPTER TWO
[1]George Watson, Ph.D., *Nutrition and Your Mind* (New York: Harper & Row, 1972), p. 150.
[2]C. L. Derrick, *Oxford Looseleaf Medicine*, IV, 178 (28), p. 12.
[3]David Hawkins and Linus Pauling, *Orthomolecular Psychiatry* (San Francisco: W. H. Freeman, 1973), p. 31.

CHAPTER THREE
[1]Abraham Hoffer, M.D., *How to Live with Schizophrenia* (New Hyde Park, N.Y.: University Books, 1966), p. 49.
[2]E. M. Abrahamson, M.D., and A. W. Pezet, *Body, Mind and Sugar* (New York: Pyramid Books, 1975), p. 120.
[3]Carlton Fredericks, Ph.D., and Herman Goodman, M.D., *Low Blood Sugar and You* (New York: Grosset & Dunlap, 1969), p. 4.

CHAPTER FOUR
[1]Gena Larson, *Better Food for Better Babies* (New Canaan, Conn.: Keats Publishing, Inc., 1972), p. 5.

CHAPTER SIX
[1]Philip S. Chen, Ph.D., with Helen D. Chung, M.S., *Soybeans for Health and a Longer Life* (New Canaan, Conn.: Keats Publishing, Inc., 1973), p. 26.
[2]*Ibid.*, p. 30.
[3]George Dock, Jr., *Harper's Magazine.* Condensed by *The Reader's Digest,* November 1946.

CHAPTER SEVEN
[1]*The Rodale Herb Book* (Emmaus, Pa.: Rodale Press, 1974).

CHAPTER EIGHT
[1]Tom R. Blaine, *Goodbye Allergies* (Secaucus, N.J.: Citadel Press, 1965).

CHAPTER NINE
[1]Bruce W. Halstead, M.D., *Chelation Therapy* (Loma Linda, Calif.: Life and Health Medical Group, 1974).

CHAPTER TEN
[1]Arthur Wallis, *God's Chosen Fast* (Christian Literature Crusade, 1969), p. 9.
[2]Allan Cott, *Fasting: The Ultimate Diet* (New York: Bantam Books, 1975).
[3]Paavo O. Airola, *How to Keep Slim, Healthy, and Young with Juice Fasting* (Phoenix: Health Plus Publishers).

CHAPTER TWELVE
[1]Kenneth H. Cooper, *Aerobics* (M. Evans Co., 1973).

BIBLIOGRAPHY

Abrahamson, E. M., and Pezet, A. W. *Body, Mind & Sugar.* New York: Pyramid, 1951.

Blaine, Tom R. *Goodbye Allergies.* Secaucus, N.J.: Citadel Press, 1965.

_____. *Mental Health Through Nutrition.* New York: N.Y. 1969.

Chen, Philip S., and Chung, Helen D. *Soybeans for Health and a Longer Life.* New Canaan, Conn.: Keats Publishing, 1973.

Cheraskin, E., and Ringsdorft, W. M., Jr. *Psycho Dietetics.* New York: Stein and Day, 1974.

Clark, Linda. *Know Your Nutrition.* New Canaan, Conn.: Keats Publishing, Inc., 1973.

Cleave, T. L. *The Saccharine Disease.* New Canaan, Conn.: Keats Publishing, Inc., 1974.

Coca, Arthur F. *The Pulse Test, Easy Allergy Detection.* New York: Arco Publishing, 1972.

Cott, Allan. *Fasting: The Ultimate Diet.* New York: Bantam Books, 1975.

Dankenbring, William F. *Your Keys to Radiant Health.* New Canaan, Conn.: Keats Publishing, Inc., 1974.

Davis, Adelle. *Let's Eat Right to Keep Fit.* New York: Harcourt Brace Jovanovich, 1970.

DiCyan, Erwin. *Vitamins in Your Life.* New York: Simon and Schuster, 1974.

Hunter, Beatrice Trum. *Fact Book on Food Additives and Your Health.* New Canaan, Conn.: Keats Publishing, Inc., 1972.

_____. *Yogurt, Kefir and Other Milk Cultures.* New Canaan, Conn.: Keats Publishing, Inc., 1973.

Hylton, William H. *The Rodale Herb Book.* Emmaus, Pa.: Rodale Press, 1974.

Harvis, D. C. *Folk Medicine.* Greenwich, Conn.: Fawcett Publications, 1958.

Jones, Dorothea Van Gundy. *The Soybean Cookbook.* New York: Arco Publishing, 1974.

Kugler, Hans J. *Slowing Down the Aging Process.* New York: Pyramid Books, 1973.

La Leche League. *The Womanly Art of Breastfeeding.* Oak Park, Ill., 1971.

Lappé, Francis Moore. *Diet for a Small Planet.* New York: Ballantine Books, 1975.

Larson, Gena. *Better Food for Better Babies and Their Families.* New Canaan, Conn.: Keats Publishing, Inc., 1972.

Martin, Clement G. *Low Blood Sugar, The Hidden Menace of Hypoglycemia.* New York: Arco Publishing, 1974.

Nittler, Alan H. *A New Breed of Doctor.* New York: Pyramid Books, 1972.

Page, Melvin E., and Abrams, H. Leon Jr. *Your Body Is Your Best Doctor!* New Canaan, Conn.: Keats Publishing, Inc., 1972.

Paterson, Grusha D., Editor. *Health's-a-Poppin'.* New York: Pyramid Books, 1973.

Pinckney, Edward R., and Pinckney, Cathey. *The Cholesterol Controversy.* Los Angeles: Sherbourne Press, 1973.

Ratcliffe, J. D. *Your Body and How It Works.* Pleasantville, N.Y.: Reader's Digest Press/Delacorte Press, 1974.

Schroeder, Henry A. *The Trace Elements and Man.* Old Greenwich, Conn.: The Devin-Adair Co., 1973.

Selye, Hans. *The Stress of Life.* New York: McGraw-Hill, 1956.

Shute, Wilfrid E., and Taub, Harald J. *Vitamin E for Ailing and Healthy Hearts.* New York: Pyramid Books, 1969.

Stone, Irwin. *The Healing Factor, Vitamin C Against Disease.* New York: Grosset & Dunlap, 1974.

Suttie, John W. *Introduction to Biochemistry.* New York: Holt, Rinehart and Winston, 1972.

Verrett, Jacqueline, and Carper, Jean. *Eating May Be Hazardous to Your Health.* New York: Doubleday Anchor Books, 1975.

Wade, Carlson. *Fats, Oils and Cholesterol.* New Canaan, Conn.: Keats Publishing, Inc., 1973.

———. *Hypertension (High Blood Pressure) and Your Diet.* New Canaan, Conn.: Keats Publishing Co., Inc., 1975.

———. *Vitamins and Other Food Supplements and Your Health.* New Canaan, Conn.: Keats Publishing, Inc., 1974.

Walczak, Michael, Editor. *Nutrition–Applied Personally.* La Habra, Calif.: International College of Applied Nutrition, 1973.

Wallis, Arthur. *God's Chosen Fast.* Fort Washington, Pa.: Christian Literature Crusade, 1969.

Watson, George. *Nutrition and Your Mind.* New York: Harper & Row, 1972.

Williams, Roger J. *Nutrition in a Nutshell.* New York: Doubleday, 1962.

Williams, Roger J. *You Are Extraordinary.* New York: Pyramid Books, 1974.

INDEX